Hospital Enterprises Management

Hospital Enterprises Management

C.Charles

ANMOL PUBLICATIONS PVT. LTD.
NEW DELHI - 110 002 (INDIA)

ANMOL PUBLICATIONS PVT. LTD.
H.O.: 4374/4B, Ansari Road, Darya Ganj
New Delhi-110 002 (India)
Ph.: 23278000, 23261597
B.O.: 1015, Ist Main Road, BSK IIIrd Stage
IIIrd Phase, IIIrd Block
Bangalore - 560 085 (Karnataka)
Ph: 080-41723429, Tel/Fax: 080-2672 3604
Visit us at: www.anmolpublications.com

Hospital Enterprises Management

First Published, 2008

ISBN 978-81-261-3285-0

PRINTED IN INDIA

Printed at Mehra Offset Press, Delhi.

Contents

Preface

Hospital enterprise management relates to improvement in standards of health through better management of health care and related programs. It seeks to accomplish this through management research, training, consultation and institutional networking in a national and global perspective. So hospital management involves everything from planning, finance, personnel management, purchase and supply and building maintenance to organization of laundry, catering and cleaning. Hospital/healthcare management aims at efficiency as well as cost-effectiveness at all levels of health services. The governing board, assisted by the administration, determines hospital objectives and policies. These are linked to the various departments and services. Certain must-have qualities for candidates aiming at hospital management are time management skills, personal commitment, and above all, the ability to make difficult decisions. In a way, hospital management is a great deal like hotel management, what with all the planning organizing and coordinating of services. Like the hotel manager, the hospital manager must ensure the smooth running of everyday functions such as front office, reception, billing, security, finance, marketing, customer relations, food and beverages, laundry and housekeeping. Also, these people should've a fair understanding of finance and information systems, interpretation of data apart from maintaining good communication with the staff of various departments.

Monitoring and improvement of patient care should be on a hospital manager's 'to-do' list.

In this book titled "Hospital Enterprises Management", after introducing the context in which health systems exist in developing as well as in industrialized countries, the role that hospitals are expected to play as 'enterprises' are discussed. The rationale behind such a role is explored and the experience so far available discussed. Evidence from several developing countries suggests caution and trends to discourage radical and indiscriminate introduction of market-oriented reforms, which international donors seem to be spearheading in Africa's health systems. It is likely however, that a limited, gradual introduction of selected elements of these reforms (such as some aspects of contracting out, managerial decentralization, the split between purchasing and providing functions) may find its place and eventually have a positive impact on the performance of the health systems. But 'mystique of markets' must not be allowed to deprive public hospitals of the sense of social utility and of the caring ethos which are essential requisites of a meaningful and effective public health system. In most countries outside of North America nearly all hospitals are owned and operated by the government. In Great Britain, except for a small number run by religious orders or serving special groups, most hospitals are within the National Health Service. The local hospital management committee answers directly to the regional hospital board. An electronic management in a hospital or a nursing home would require to very precise and must result into cost cutting and efficient management. Main modules of hospital management system Include:

— Patient Registration

— Appointment Scheduling

— Admission Discharge Transfer
— Bed Management
— Wards Management Module
— Patient Relations
— Doctors Workbench
— Nursing Workbench
— Operation Theater
— Electronic Medical Record
— Clinic Specialties
— Laboratory Information System
— Radiology Information System
— Pharmacy
— Central Sterilized Supply Department
— Blood Bank
— Dietary (F&B)
— Housekeeping/Laundry
— Equipment Maintenance System (EMS)
— Healthcare Packages
— Patient Billing
— Insurance and Contracts Management
— Management Information System (MIS)
— Hospital Administration
— Roster Management
— HRMS
— Financial Accounting

The objective of this book is to provide readers / students with an integrated understanding of the subject area of hospital enterprise management.

—Editor

1

Introduction to Hospital Organisation and Patient Care Quality

HOSPITAL ORGANISATION AND QUALITY OF PATIENT CARE

Some hospital trusts and health authorities consistently outperform others on different dimensions of performance. Why? There is some evidence that "management matters", as well as the combined efforts of individual clinicians and teams. However, studies that have been conducted on the link between the organisation and management of services and quality of patient care can be criticised both theoretically and methodologically. A larger, and arguably more rigorous, body of work exists on the performance of firms in the private sector, often conducted within the disciplines of organisational behaviour or human resource management. Studies in these traditions have focused on the effects of decentralisation, participation, innovative work practices, and "complementarities" on outcome variables such as job satisfaction and performance. The aim of this paper is to identify a number of reviews and research traditions that might bring new ideas into future work on the determinants of hospital performance. Ideally, future research should be more theoretically informed and should use longitudinal rather than cross sectional research designs. The use of statistical methods such as multilevel modelling, which allow for the inclusion of variables at different levels of analysis, would enable estimation of the separate contribution that, structure and process make to hospital outcomes.

Organisational researchers have long sought to establish the impact of organisational structures and managerial processes on outcomes such as profitability, effectiveness, performance, and organisational growth and survival. Organisational researchers have also focused on the public sector, particularly hospitals, in an effort to link organisational characteristics to a number of important outcomes for patients and staff. Although few would now question that "management matters" in delivering quality health care, knowledge about the nature of the relationship is incomplete. The fact that we know so little about the relationship between structures, processes, and outcomes within hospitals makes it difficult to recommend, on the basis of sound theory and empirical evidence, ways of organising that could improve patient care.

One of the criticisms of research on hospital performance is that it has been rather insular, paying little attention to developments in related fields such as organisational sociology, organisational behaviour, management studies, or human resource management. Most of these disciplines study organisational performance in the context of a market and their dependent variables are usually profitability, productivity, or market share which are very different from many of the proxies for quality of care—such as mortality or morbidity—used in studies of hospital performance. However, these reports are similarly concerned with issues of motivating, engaging, and rewarding staff which may be linked to patient outcomes as well as to business success. Greater attention to the work that has been done on organisational performance, broadly defined, could illuminate our attempts to link the characteristics of hospitals and units to the kind of care they are able to provide to patients.

Of course, the disciplines of organisational sociology and human resource management are vast and the aims of this paper are modest. It is impossible to treat the literature on these subjects in great depth here. The main aim of this paper is to identify a number of "landmark studies", defined as frequently cited review articles, that try to make sense of the burgeoning literature on organisational performance. These studies could contribute to the development of theory in this area. A second aim is to identify variables at different levels of analysis—individual, organisational, and environmental—that could be used in future models of hospital organisation and quality of patient care.

Key Messages

— Studies linking the organisation and management of health care to patient and staff outcomes, mainly conducted in the USA, can be criticised both theoretically and methodologically.

— There are currently no high quality studies of these relationships in the UK.

— This paper identifies key review articles of studies, both in health care and in business, that might throw new light on the determinants of hospital performance.

— Research on the performance of business firms suggests the importance of decentralised decision making, staff participation and involvement, innovative work practices, and the "fit" between structure, strategy, and environment.

Future research could be improved by greater attention to the mechanisms that might plausibly link, for example, staff variables to patient outcomes by adopting longitudinal rather than cross sectional research designs and by using appropriate statistical methods such as multilevel modelling.

Health Policies Motivating Organisational Research

The message from the current UK government that quality of care must be given greater priority than in the past has been widely welcomed by the professions. Some of the main policy documents relating to quality of care in the UK National Health Service are described. Within the quality initiative there is a clear recognition that only so much can be achieved by appealing to individual practitioners, and that more effort needs to be expended on understanding how the organisation and management of care affects outcomes. Many of the goals of the new NHS—including clearer lines of accountability and responsibility, better communication, and improved conditions for staff—require interventions at the level of the organisation.

One of the most important planks in the quality platform is the policy of clinical governance. Clinical governance has been defined as "a framework through which NHS organisations are accountable for continuously improving the quality of their services and safeguarding high standards of care by creating an environment in which excellence in clinical care can flourish". Buetow and Roland noted that the "duty of quality" relates to the organisation, not just to individuals within the organisation. Although a named individual, most often the Chief Executive, will assume statutory responsibility for quality, many trusts have already implemented structural changes, creating new layers of management and establishing new committees to enable them to meet the challenge of clinical governance. Clinical governance also demands cultural change towards openness, participation, staff empowerment, partnership, and collaboration; an important goal is to move away from a culture based on blame to one that emphasises learning from mistakes. The emphasis on the need for structural and cultural change in both organisations and professions recognises that not all the quality goals of the NHS can be achieved by inducing or exhorting individual clinicians and managers to change their own practice.

The quality of patient care may be related in an important way to the quality of life experienced by staff at work. Partly as a result of the quality initiative, concern about the way the NHS treats its employees has increased. Issues of human resource management have also been highlighted by the projected crisis in the number of nurses and by the dissatisfaction of junior doctors with their working hours. Too few trained nurses, combined with overworked and fatigued doctors, are not a recipe for excellence in patient care. So, how can we improve the quality of working life in ways that will enhance the ability of the NHS to recruit and retain staff? Pay, flexible hours, and job prospects are obviously central, but improving the quality of working life also means helping individuals to develop their potential, to increase their sense of autonomy, and the ability to achieve their goals. At the same time, attention needs to focus on organisational development. Creating an environment that is perceived as "a good place to work" requires multiple interventions at different levels. Clinical governance and better human resource management practices are important planks in the current health policies emphasising quality of patient care. Both planks demand attention, not just to the individual level of analysis, but to the ways that clinical directorates, divisions, trust boards, and professions work together to achieve quality. These goals move organisational research onto the centre stage.

Organisation of Nursing Work

In the early 1980s the American Nurses' Association identified a group of hospitals that were known by reputation as "good places to work". Designated as "magnet" hospitals because they had little difficulty in recruiting and retaining staff, they were found to share a number of organisational features, including:

- a relatively flat nursing hierarchy with few supervisors;
- the chief nurse had a strong position in the management structure of the hospital;
- nurses had autonomy to make clinical decisions in their own areas of competence and had control over their own practice;
- decision making was decentralised at the level of the unit;
- staffing was adequate and limits were placed on the number of new nursing graduates;
- methods to facilitate communication between nurses and physicians were established;
- the organisation of nurses' work promoted accountability and continuity of care—for example, primary nursing care;
- the institution demonstrated the value it attached to nurses—for example, by investing in their education.

Aiken and colleagues at the University of Pennsylvania have since shown in a series of studies that cardinal features of the "magnet" hospitals are related to lower mortality rates, increased patient satisfaction, and lower burnout rates and needle stick injuries among nursing staff. These methodologically sophisticated studies use a research strategy whereby data gathered from individuals about their sense of autonomy, control over their own work, and quality of communication are aggregated to describe important characteristics of the organisation. This enables the researchers to estimate the relationship between structural characteristics of the organisation and outcomes for patients and staff. This research programme has now expanded to include an international sample including hospitals and nurses in Scotland and England. The results of this study, which is currently underway, will have much potential to inform policies for changing the organisation of nursing work to promote positive patient outcomes.

Organisational Research Focusing on Hospitals

Studies of the organisation and management of hospitals have examined the impact of a dizzying array of factors on the quality of patient care. Flood, in a wide ranging review of organisational research conducted mainly in the USA in the 1980s, identified the basic sources of variation that were found to be associated with quality of patient care.

A number of studies have found a weak relationship between doctors' training and experience and quality of care. Flood has interpreted this to mean "... not that physicians are unimportant for quality but that organisational context is far more important in setting limits (upper and lower) for physicians than formerly recognised ....". Medical staff organisation—including peer review, selection and continued review of new staff members, and participation in policy making committees—have also been shown to be positively related to quality of patient care.

Few studies have examined whether a similar set of relationships hold for other staff, but studies of coordination and communication have focused on nurses and ancillary staff. Coordination appears to be particularly significant, and a series of studies conducted in intensive care found that "conflict management skills, including communication, problem solving and leadership, combined with a patient orientation" were positively related to quality of patient care. Flood suggests that one promising area for future research will be the extent to which the boundary between the two traditional authority structures—professional and administrative—are breached in hospital organisations.

There is a well established relationship between the volume of patients passing through a health care unit and the quality of care delivered, although there is disagreement as to the mechanism generating this relationship. The literature proposes at least five plausible hypotheses, two of which rely on the idea that "practice makes perfect"—that is, the skills of individual practitioners are enhanced by specialisation and by repeated performance of the same or similar tasks. Highly skilled and specialised practitioners also provide better peer review. A third mechanism involves units with good reputations attracting more referrals and consequently having a high volume. It has also been suggested that high volumes are associated with a more preventative orientation among a group of doctors, with patients being treated at an earlier stage of their illness. Finally, some studies have suggested that "... volume of similar cases leads to benefits because the organisation and its staff become more practised in managing and caring for these patients or because certain efficiencies can be introduced with sufficient volume much akin to economies of scale".

Flood surmises that many different mechanisms may be operating at once to produce the relationship between volume and quality, but it is clear that extent of specialisation of staff, volume of patients, and case mix are important variables in relation to quality of patient care. Complexity can take many forms—for example, the severity of each individual patient's illness, the frequency of multiple diagnoses, and the number of patients who have combined health and social problems—which require the coordination of a large number of clinicians and services. It also includes characteristics of the work, such as whether or not admission patterns are predictable. Complexity could plausibly be related to quality of care and contingency theory would suggest that some managerial approaches will work for some groups of patients and types of services and not for others.

A number of stable characteristics of hospitals have also been related to outcomes. One consistent finding is that quality of care is better in hospitals affiliated to a major medical school. Findings over the last 30 years have shown, at least in the USA, that teaching hospitals affiliated to a major medical school tend to be associated with higher costs, better quality outcomes, and more sophisticated techniques, after taking into account patient mix.

Flood concluded from her review of studies of health care organisations that, although much of this research can be criticised both theoretically and methodologically, there is at least some support for the relationship between quality of care and a number of variables. The most serious deficiencies in this body of research lie in the failure to specify the mechanism linking organisational characteristics to outcomes, and in failing to show that organisational and managerial factors come logically before quality. It is still possible to infer from many studies of this type that quality of care might have caused changes in the structure of the organisation, managerial processes, or in the kind of staff who chose to work there, rather than the other way round. Many studies also focus exclusively on the internal structure and processes of the hospital and fail to consider the wider environment, particularly the network of relationships in which hospitals operate. The omission of environmental and relational variables would be particularly egregious in models of quality in the NHS where the links between the organisation and the healthcare system are particularly important. Flood also criticises the lack of attention to culture as an important influence on managerial decision making. Future research should try to make some theoretical progress in this area which will help to explain how organisational structures and processes, as well as the internal and external environments, are related to quality of care. The problem of causal ordering, which is ubiquitous in organisational research, can only really be addressed by longitudinal rather than by cross sectional research designs.

Whereas Flood focused her review on the independent variables, a recent review has examined the variety of dependent variables that are frequently used in studies of hospital performance. Mitchell and Shortell set out to examine "the state of the science with respect to morbidity, mortality and adverse events indicative of organisational variables in care delivery systems". They found a total of 81 studies in this area, most of which were conducted in acute care settings in the USA during the 1990s. The independent variables in these studies were more frequently features of the organisational structure (high technology, nurse staffing, professional expertise, size, ownership, urban/rural location, teaching hospital status) than organisational or clinical processes (collaboration and care coordination, volume of patients).

In general, they found that this body of work provides some support for the conclusion that nursing surveillance, quality of working environment, and quality of interaction among professionals distinguish hospitals with lower mortality and complications from those with higher rates of adverse events. However, empirical results are ambiguous.

As researchers become increasingly adept at controlling for patient factors such as severity of illness, the organisation and managerial variables tend to decrease in significance.

The main contribution of this review is the fact that they distinguish between the different kinds of dependent variables—mortality, complications (surgical complications, infections), and other adverse events (falls, pressure sores, and medication errors). They show that these three are not interchangeable and suggest that there are problems in using each as a proxy for quality of care. The authors argue that mortality and adverse events are important outcome measures because they can alert us when things are going badly wrong in a healthcare setting. However, if we want to understand how the organisation and management of hospitals affects patient outcomes, mortality in particular may not be the best dependent variable because death rates are so heavily dependent on patient characteristics.

Mitchell and Shortell suggest that "... given that adverse events appear more closely related to organisational factors than to mortality, researchers need to refine and better define such events that are logically related to the co-ordinative organisational processes among caregivers." The "failure to rescue" measure developed by Silber *et al* is a significant development in this area. This conditional probability—death rates following complications—has been found to be more closely related to hospital factors than raw mortality figures. The idea is that, while the likelihood that a patient will develop a complication is largely due to factors such as their age and severity of illness, the likelihood that they survive following development of a complication is at least partly a function of the care they receive. Finally, Mitchell and Shortell recommend that future research should focus on smaller care giving units rather than on the hospital because units within a hospital vary greatly.

Using the hospital as the unit of analysis may be masking the effect of organisational and managerial variables as the amount of variation within a hospital may be greater than that which exists between hospitals.

Research on Non-Hospital Organisations

Although there are many differences between hospitals and other kinds of organisations such as business firms and industries, research on organisational outcomes provides support for some of the independent variables identified by Flood and Aiken and suggests some additional variables that might be considered. Clues from the literature on industry, firms, and other businesses suggest that decentralisation and participation in management, which are organisational level variables related to autonomy and control at the individual level, should be considered as contenders for a place in a causal model. Some of these variables refer to organisational structures and others to processes, and these will be discussed in turn. Mintzberg explains the importance of structure in the following way: "Every organised human activity—from the making of pots to placing a man on the moon—gives rise to two fundamental and opposing requirements: the division of labour into various tasks to be performed, and the coordination of these tasks to accomplish the activity.

The structure of an organisation can be defined simply as the sum total of the ways in which it divides its labour into distinct tasks and then achieves coordination among them." Most standard texts in management studies have at least one chapter on organisational structures. Dawson, for example, in a chapter entitled "Coordination and control: structure and organisational design" defines organisational structure as "... the socially created pattern of rules, roles and relationships that exist within [the organisation]." In contrast, the culture of an organisation refers to the collection of values and beliefs within it.

Mintzberg implies that there is a strong relationship between culture and structure. His classification of organisational *configurations* suggests, for example, that organisations with relatively non-hierarchical structures such as universities are likely to have very different cultures from organisations such as the army that have a strong hierarchical structure. One of the most interesting features of an organisational structure is the extent to which it is centralised or decentralised. According to Simon *et al* : "An administrative organisation is centralised to the extent that decisions are made at relatively high levels in the organisation; decentralised to the extent that discretion and authority to make important decisions are delegated by top management to lower levels of executive authority". The two concepts are not mirror images; some empirical work suggests that they are, in fact, weakly correlated. Studies also suggest that there are at least two separate notions embedded in the concept of decentralisation, the first referring to the hierarchical levels at which decisions are made (or influenced) and the second referring to the extent to which different levels participate in the decision making process.

These arguments suggest that both centralisation and decentralisation should be seen as multidimensional concepts. Traditionally, centralisation is measured in two main ways. Pugh *et al*, who pioneered the examination of organisational structures, collected data on, for example, the Chief Executive's span of control and the ratio of workers to supervisors, mainly from documentary evidence collected from organisations. Hage and Aiken focused on participation in decision making and hierarchy of authority. In their landmark study of centralisation these authors interviewed staff in 16 social welfare and health organisations in the USA where they focused on behaviour—particularly participation in hiring, promotion, policies, and programmes—as well as the extent to which each individual felt he or she had to defer to a supervisor. Although both of these measures have been well used in organisational research, we might question whether either would provide an adequate measure of decentralisation in the NHS in the UK.

Acorn *et al* used Hage and Aiken's instrument to survey acute care nurse managers in a recent US study. The dependent variables of interest were autonomy, job satisfaction, and commitment to the organisation. Scores on decentralisation were not normally distributed because, the authors argue, most hospitals in the USA are decentralised to some degree, and were recoded as a trichotomous variable. Path analysis showed that decentralisation produced significant positive effects on autonomy, job satisfaction, and organisational commitment, and influenced commitment through autonomy and job satisfaction.

Decentralisation is related to the notion of "participative management" which is widely used in organisational behaviour and management studies. Wagner defines participation as "... a process in which influence is shared among individuals who are otherwise hierarchical unequals". Participative management practices mean the involvement of managers and subordinates in information processing, decision making, and problem solving. Cotton *et al* identified 68 studies of participation but found that there were some important differences in the way researchers defined the key term. In order to analyse the effects of different forms of participation they classified studies into six groups depending on the focus of the study, as shown as:

Organisational and Managerial Factors Related to Organisational Performance

- Leadership and management skills
- Clear organisational objectives and strategies for achieving them
- The "fit" between organisational objectives, external environment, and strategy
- Change management processes
- An organisational culture that is receptive to change and good working relationships among key actors
- Good relationships between separate parts of the NHS network with clarity over "who does what"
- Use of performance management, supported by good information systems, to drive change
- Recognition that "good performance" is multidimensional and that the components of performance, such as quality of care and financial success, are not necessarily competitive

Pettigrew *et al* criticised this work for the historical tendency to focus on one determinant of quality such as human resource management practices, rather than attempting to construct and estimate multivariate models. In some ways the idea of "bundling" can be seen as an attempt to redress the balance in favour of more complex models. These authors identified the recent theoretical writings of industrial economists Milgrom and Roberts as an important impetus to future work in this area. The complementarities approach argues that sets of factors can be mutually reinforcing in their effects on performance. Their recommendation is that future research on the performance of healthcare institutions should, at least in part, use the idea of complementarities.

Towards a model of the organisational impacts on quality of patient care

The aim of this paper has been to identify, from the literature, some of the organisational variables that might belong in a model of quality of care. These appear to fall into a number of categories which are summarised as:

Types of Variables that Might be Included in Modelling Organisational Outcomes

Independent Variables

— Organisational structures, e.g. decentralisation

— Organisational processes, e.g. human resource management practices, coordination of care, interprofessional relationships

— Environmental variables, e.g. quality of relationships with other organisations

— Social psychology of work, e.g. individuals' experience of participation in decision making, sense of autonomy, and control

— "Fit" among strategy, structure, and environment

Intermediate Variables

— Staff outcomes, e.g. job satisfaction

— Organisational outcomes, e.g. rate of sickness and absenteeism

Control Variables

— Hospital characteristics, e.g. size, specialisation, teaching status, number of staff

— Patient characteristics, e.g. severity of illness, multiple diagnoses

— Characteristics of work, e.g. predictability of admission patterns, volume

— Socioeconomic factors, e.g. social class characteristics of local population, urban/rural location
— Economic variables, e.g. financial state of the organisation

Dependent Variables

— Clinical indicators, e.g. deaths in hospital within 30 days of admission
— Adverse events, e.g. medication errors, falls
— Complications, e.g. hospital acquired infections
— Constructed indicators, e.g. failure to rescue
— Administrative targets, e.g. state of waiting lists, financial viability
— Patients and carers' experiences, e.g. complaints, response to surveys

Structural features of the organisation might include the extent to which the organisation is centralised or decentralised, which can be measured either as the level at which decisions are taken or by the number of levels in the hierarchy. The ratio of supervisory to non-supervisory positions is a crude measure of centralisation. NHS hospitals also differ in the extent to which departments such as finance or personnel are devolved out of their own professional departments into management teams. The extent to which clinicians are involved in management also seems to be an important distinguishing feature of some current NHS trusts, which might have important implications for sharing power and responsibility.

Organisational processes, such as innovative human resource management practices and procedures to facilitate communication, conflict resolution, and participation are also important. Both of these categories are at the organisational level of analysis because neither set of variables is reducible to the behaviour of individuals. They are therefore logically prior to the *social psychological* variables that describe the experience of working in a particular place.

In this category the literature stresses the relationship between participation in decision making, sense of involvement in the organisation, and sense of autonomy and control. Taken together, the structural features of the organisation and the processes it employs partially determine the subjective experiences of workers (*staff outcomes*) such as job satisfaction and morale, and contribute to *organisational outcomes* such as difficulties in recruiting and retaining staff.

The main variable that we want to explain is *quality of patient care* which could be estimated, in the first instance, by using the NHS performance indicators published for England in 1999 and 2000. These could also be used to calculate more theoretically defensible dependent variables such as the "failure to rescue" measure described by Silber *et al*. We also need to consider a number of *control variables.* These are variables which have been shown to have a significant association with quality—for example, size, teaching status, extent of specialisation, staff number and skill mix, and the volume and case mix of patients.

This group of variables would also include human capital variables such as the training, education and experience of staff, or tenure in the case of the top management team. Finally, having criticised previous research for omitting environmental variables, we could include some measures of the extent to which the organisation is influenced or controlled by external forces and the quality of relationships they enjoy with other organisations.

Different Types of Participation

— Participation in work decisions: permanent programmes where workers take a formal direct role in decisions about their work

— Consultative participation: long term interventions such as quality circles where employees are consulted as managers make decisions

— Short term participation: brief but formal exercises in participatory decision making about job issues

— Informal participation: managers and subordinates engage in informal influence sharing despite the absence of a formal programme

— Employee ownership

— Representative participation: employees are elected as council or board members

Cotton *et al* then showed that not all forms of participation are equally effective. The "winners" appear to be participation in work decisions, informal participation (which was associated primarily with enhanced job performance), and employee ownership (associated with enhanced job satisfaction). We might speculate that participation appears to be most effective when it is a permanent and inclusive feature of the employment relation rather than sporadic or exclusive. This would explain why consultative, short term, and representative participation—which are either episodic or involve only selected individuals rather than all employees—appear to have less impact on performance and job satisfaction than other more consistent forms of participation.

The significance and cost effectiveness of participative management have been the subjects of some debate in management studies. The literature seems to suggest that participation has some beneficial effects, but is it worth the costs of reorganisation and training of staff that would be involved in implementation? To establish the current state of knowledge Wagner examined 10 meta-analyses which focused on the effects of participation on job satisfaction and performance. The author excluded from the review studies of delegation where managers relinquished all influence to their subordinates, studies of consultation where subordinates were involved in idea generation but were not involved in selecting the final idea, and more comprehensive and extensive programmes, such as job enrichment interventions and quality of work life programmes. He concluded that current evidence is consistent with the claim that participation has a statistically significant positive effect on job performance and satisfaction but that the actual effects are limited in size. In practical terms, this leaves unanswered the question of whether the high costs associated with introducing participation in management are justified. If, as Wagner suggests might be the case, the effect of participation is cumulative, with "small episodic influences" building over time, then it may indeed be a good strategy for an organisation to pursue. Current research, which is predominantly cross sectional, may miss changes that occur over time.

Decentralisation and participative management are related to a number of other "innovative work practices" which have been reviewed by Ichniowski *et al.* Within this broad term they include efforts to improve workers' involvement (such as profit sharing, flexible and broadly defined work assignments), improved communication and dispute resolution mechanisms, and worker participation in decision making. These can be contrasted with traditional work practices where jobs have clear boundaries and associated rates of pay, where there are clear lines between workers and supervisors, decisions are made almost exclusively by managers, and communication flows through the formal chain of command. They concluded that: "Innovative human resource management practices can improve business productivity, primarily through the use of systems of related work practices designed to enhance worker participation and flexibility in the design of work and decentralisation of management tasks and responsibilities". They also suggested that there are potentially large payoffs—that is, the consequences of adopting participative work practices can have economically important effects on the performance of firms that adopt them. Perhaps the most important finding is that the *specific* work practice is less effective than the co-existence of a number of similar practices that improve productivity and attitudes as well as decrease turnover and accidents. This is the phenomenon of "bundling", which is used to describe the combination of high involvement work practices and supporting management practices. "Workers cannot make good decisions without sufficient information and training, and they are unlikely to make suggestions if they feel that this will cost them their jobs or reduce their pay". It is tempting to conclude that some underlying cultural shift in the relationship between workers and managers is a necessary prerequisite for beneficial changes in the structure and functioning of the organisation. In other words, tinkering with one or two organisational innovations is not enough. The question of the extent to which high involvement work practices and supporting management practices have been adopted in the NHS has still to be determined. However, if trusts do vary on these dimensions, it makes an empirical test of the relationship between work practices and quality of care at least theoretically possible.

Similar conclusions emerged from a review of the

literature on the determinants of organisational performance commissioned by the National Health Service Executive and conducted by Pettigrew and colleagues at Warwick and Aston Business Schools. They were asked to identify and synthesise what is known and not known about the determinants of performance in private and public sector organisations, and about the practices and techniques of performance management. They found there is more literature on performance measurement, less on performance management, and least on the determinants of performance. Relative to research on the private sector, research on the determinants of public sector performance is very limited in quality as well as quantity. In fact, they could find no quality studies of the determinants of performance in trusts. They concluded that the most comprehensive, illuminating, and useful research on performance determinants in healthcare settings has been carried out in the USA by Shortell and colleagues. This work, which was mainly conducted on managed care organisations, raises important findings and questions for the implementation of primary care groups. There is some evidence—for example, in the work by Shortell *et al*, Pettigrew, and Collins and Porras —for the impact of a number of organisational and managerial factors that are related to organisational performance in both the public and private sectors.

Taking this Work Forward

Understanding how the organisation and management of hospitals affects the quality of patient care is no mean task. Previous research can help us to identify some of the variables that appear to be relevant, but we do not yet have a theory that reflects the complexity of the relationships involved. This paper, by drawing on a number of different fields of literature, has sought to identify variables at different levels of analysis—individual, organisational, and environmental—that might be linked. The next step will be to articulate how they might be related to each other and to build simple models that will guide empirical investigation. This will entail dealing with issues such as causal ordering, identification of mechanisms, and specification of temporal sequences that have dogged this tradition of research for many years. Ideally, future research will be more theoretically informed, will use longitudinal rather than cross sectional research designs (so that the problem of causal ordering can be addressed), and will use statistical methods such as multilevel modelling which allow for the inclusion of variables at different levels of analysis.

A great deal of research is currently underway that will strengthen the evidence on which recommendations about the organisation and management of hospitals can be based. However, the process of producing good quality research can be prolonged. In the meantime, it is important to communicate the importance of organisational factors to clinicians, to whom they may be relatively unknown. Medical and nursing education tends to focus, quite rightly, on individual patient care, and an awareness of how each clinical encounter is constrained or enabled by the system within which it is embedded can take many years of clinical practice. We all need to become much more conscious of how the way we work together, and the way that care is organised, affects patients' experience of the healthcare system.

CONSULTATIONS AND SPECIAL SERVICES

The AMA CPT manual defines a consultation as a type of service provided by a physician whose opinion or advice regarding evaluation and/or management of a specific problem is requested by another physician or other appropriate source.

There are four subcategories of consultations: *office (outpatient), initial inpatient, follow-up inpatient* and *confirmatory*. Office or other outpatient consultation codes (99241-99245) and confirmatory consultation codes (99271-99275) are discussed in this chapter. Initial inpatient and follow-up inpatient consultations are discussed.

The difference between consultations and new patient visits is often a source of confusion. The difference in reimbursement is sometimes dramatic, so it is important for rheumatologists to understand the distinction.

The Medicare Carrier Manual provides some insight on this issue. Consultations must meet the criteria for a particular consultation code.. The request for a consultation from the attending physician or other appropriate source, and the need for consultation must be documented in the patient's medical record. The consultant's opinion and any services that were ordered or performed must also be documented in the patient's medical record and communicated to the requesting physician or other appropriate source. For documentation purposes, a written request from the referring physician should be included in the patient's medical record, or the consulting physician's records should show a specific reference to the request.

A consultant may initiate diagnostic and/or therapeutic services at the initial consultation without losing consultant status. If the rheumatologist consultant subsequently assumes responsibility for management of a portion or all of the patient's condition, the established patient office visit codes (99211-99215) must be used for follow-up visits. Note that there are no codes for follow-up consultations, except in the context of inpatient care. Also, note that Medicare carriers interpret national policies in different ways, particularly related to the initiation of therapeutic services. If you have questions, you should direct them to your carrier.

If an additional request for opinion or advice regarding the same or a new problem is received from the attending physician and documented in the medical record, the office consultation codes (99241-99245) may be reported again by the rheumatologist consultant.

A "consultation" initiated by a non-physician (patient, patient's family, third party payor, etc.) for a second or third opinion is reported using the confirmatory consultation codes (99271-99275) or the new patient office visit codes (99201-99205), as appropriate. If the confirmatory consultation is required by a third party payor, then the modifier "-32" or 09932 (mandated services), should be added to the appropriate confirmatory consultation code. Any specifically identifiable procedure (e.g., identified with a specific CPT code) performed on or subsequent to the date of the initial consultation should be reported separately.

For definitions of the levels of E/M services. Like new patient and established patient office visits, office or other outpatient consultations have five levels of services recognized by the CPT codes. The descriptions for each level of service in this chapter are taken from the AMA CPT manual. Each level of service is followed by a patient encounter example. Some of the patient examples have been validated by the AMA; however, many of the examples have not been validated and are, therefore, subject to change. Only those examples labeled "AMA/CPT validated example" have gone through the AMA validation process.

Nursing Facility, Domiciliary, Rest Home, Custodial Care and Home Services

There are CPT codes to describe the care provided for new or established patients in facilities outside of the hospital.

Nursing Facilities (formerly called skilled nursing facilities, intermediate care facilities and long-term care facilities) are reported using the "Nursing Facility Services" codes (CPT 99301-99313). CPT codes 99301-99303 identify comprehensive nursing facility care assessments performed at one or more sites in the assessment process: the hospital, office, nursing facility, domiciliary/non-nursing facility or patient's home. CPT codes 99311-99313 should be used to identify subsequent nursing facility care. Check with your local carriers regarding the requirements for compliance with these assessments.

Domiciliary, rest home (e.g., boarding home) or custodial care service CPT codes identify evaluation and management services in a facility which provides room, board and other personal assistance, generally on a long-term basis. The facility's services do not include a medical component. To report care delivered in such facilities, use codes 99321-99323 for a new patient and codes 99331-99333 for an established patient.

Many patients with rheumatic diseases are homebound or may occasionally be unable to visit the office. *In such situations, rheumatologists may be called to visit patients at home*. Codes 99341-99343 refer to home care for a new patient, while codes 99351-99353 refer to home care for an established patient. Please refer to the AMA's CPT manual for more specific guidelines with regard to the reporting of E/M services provided in a private residence.

Prolonged Services

CPT codes 99354-99357 are used when a physician provides prolonged service involving direct (face-to-face) patient contact that is beyond the usual service in either the inpatient or outpatient setting. This service is reported in addition to other physician services, including evaluation and management services at any level.

To report a prolonged service, the evaluation and management service provided must exceed the typical time specified in the code by at least 30 minutes. The time spent by the physician on a given date does not have to be continuous. Please note, these codes do not include time that a patient spends occupying an exam or treatment room where there is no direct physician-patient contact or time spent with a non-physician "incident to" a physician's service.

There are also CPT codes for prolonged physician services without direct (face-to-face) patient contact. Prolonged physician service CPT codes 99358 and 99359 are used when a physician provides prolonged service *not* involving direct (face-to-face) care that is beyond the usual service in either the inpatient or outpatient setting. For example, CPT codes 99358-99359 are used to report review of extensive records and tests and communication with other professionals and/or the patient/family. CPT code 99360 is used to report physician standby services. To report telephone calls, report CPT codes 99371-99373. Note: Medicare factors the work involved in telephone calls into individual E/M codes and does not reimburse separately for telephone calls. Please refer to the AMA CPT manual for more specific guidelines.

Care Plan Oversight Services

Care plan oversight services codes (CPT 99374-99380) are used to bill for physician oversight of care/therapy provided to patients in home health agencies, hospices or nursing facilities involving 30 minutes or more. Only one physician may report services within a 30-day calendar month.

For Medicare billing purposes, HCFA will allow payment for the oversight and supervision of therapy involving 30 minutes or more of the *physician's* time per calendar month if services are furnished to patients receiving Medicare-covered home health and hospice services, provided the physician has furnished a service requiring a face-to-face encounter with the patient in the six months before the first billing for the care plan oversight services; the physician does not have a significant financial relationship with the home health agency; the physician is not the medical director or employee of the hospice; and the physician does not provide services under an arrangement with the hospice.

Medicare does not cover physician supervision of nursing facility patients (CPT Codes 99379 and 99380).

Special Evaluation and Management Services

Special E/M services codes are used to report evaluations performed to establish baseline information prior to life or disability insurance certificates being issued. These services are performed in the office or other setting for both new and established patients. When using the codes, no active management of the problem(s) is undertaken during the encounter. If other evaluation and management services and/or procedures are performed on the same date, the appropriate E/M or procedure code(s) should be reported in addition to these codes. *Medicare does not reimburse for these codes.*

'Incident to' Services

"Incident to" services are furnished by a non-physician health professional as an integral yet incidental part of the physician's services. These services may not represent the major portion of the overall service provided. To be covered under Medicare's "incident to" rules, services must be:

— Commonly rendered without separate charge in the physician's bill
— Commonly furnished in the physician's office or clinic
— Furnished under the direct personal supervision of the physician
— Furnished by an employee of the physician

These rules apply to services provided by auxiliary personnel such as nurses, non-physician anesthetists, psychologists, technicians, nurse practitioners, physician's assistants and other aides, and the physician bills the services as though they were provided by the physician. Note that the physician accepts liability for all services billed in his or her name.

"Incident to" services must be directly supervised by the physician. Medicare defines this as being present in the office suite and immediately available to provide assistance and direction throughout the time the auxiliary personnel is performing services. Being available by telephone does not qualify.

If the services are provided in a patient's home or a nursing facility, direct physical supervision requires the physician to have face-to-face contact with the patient and to be in the room when the "incident to" service is rendered. The physician must be present for the duration of the service. Medicare defines "employee" as someone who is employed full-time, part-time or leased by the physician, group practice or the legal entity that employs the physician. In some instances, services can be billed either as "incident to" the physician or by the licensed practitioner (nurse practitioner, physician's assistant, clinical psychologist), but they may not be billed as both. Note that if the service is billed "incident to" the physician, all the "incident to" rules apply (physician being present, etc.) even though the licensed practitioner may legally provide the service without the physician's presence.

EMERGENCY PROCEDURES

Medical Emergencies

A. Preparedness: Students, faculty, residents and staff involved in patient services must be CPR certified. The student is advised to periodically review and mentally rehearse the steps, materials and drugs to be followed and used for a circulatory arrest emergency as presented in the course material of the Cardiopulmonary Resuscitation Course.

B. Location of Emergency Equipment: Emergency carts containing oxygen, resuscitation equipment and medications are located on each floor.

1. Third floor: Dispensary (AD-3420).
2. Second floor: Clinic 12 (AD-2311).
3. First floor: (Clinic 1, Room 1334)
4. A wheelchair is located in the Oral Surgery Clinic for emergency use.
5. An emergency action protocol is posted by each telephone in the clinics.

Oral Surgery is responsible for monthly inspection of carts to determine if they are intact and have no unexpired drugs.

Fire or Disaster Situation (Code 17)

A. Remove persons in immediate danger of the fire. Close doors to areas affected.

B. Activate the nearest fire alarm box and call PUBLIC

SAFETY DIVISION at 12911. Give the location of the fire.

C. Calmly notify other personnel in the area.

D. Attempt to extinguish the fire with the proper fire extinguisher provided in your area.

E. Follow established fire safety and evacuation procedures. Escort patients from building.

F. Remain calm. Never yell "FIRE."

Eyewash Units

Eyewash units are available in sinks throughout the school to be used in cases of contamination of the eye(s) by chemical splash, foreign objects from grinding, etc.

Clinic	*Room #*	*Area*	*Department*
1	1334	Instrument Room	Oral Surgery
3	2703	Instrument Room	Pediatric Dentistry
4*		None Available	
	2510	Wet Lab between 3,4,5,6	
5	2536	Clinical Research Instrument Room	General Practice Residency/Clinical Research
6	2631	Instrument Room	Endodontics
8	2922	Open Clinic	Orthodontics
10	2103	Supply Station	Periodontics
11*		None Available	
	2111	Wet Lab between 10, 11, 12, 13	
12	2302	Supply Station	Emergency Dental Service
13*		None Available	
14		Supply Station - Middle Bay	Oral Rehabilitation
	2009	Removable Prosthodontics Lab	Oral Rehabilitation
	3009	Fixed Restorative lab	Oral Rehabilitation
	3324	3rd Floor Preclinical Technique Lab - sink on either side (2 units)	Oral Rehabilitation

16*		None Available	
	3201	Dental Materials Lab	Dental Materials
	3202A		
17	3117	Laboratory	Oral Rehabilitation
	3136	Laboratory	
	1411B	Laboratories	Oral Biology
	1412		
	1415, 1420		
	1422, 1428		
	1431, 1432		
	1437A		
	1441A		
	1444, 1450		
	1459		

* None Available

C. Student Responsibilities

1. In case of emergency, the student should STAY WITH THE PATIENT and obtain assistance from a nearby dental assistant or from another student who can obtain the emergency cart and a supervising faculty doctor
2. Students as freshmen and again as juniors (spring semester) are required to pass a course in basic life support procedures that involves CPR certification.

Medical Emergency Protocol for the School of Dentistry

Objective

The Dental Practitioner is constantly faced with the possibility of a medical emergency during the course of patient care. He or she should, therefore, be prepared to handle such emergencies with the greatest expediency. Our plan is to instill awareness in the faculty, students and staff of the Medical Emergency Protocol and a mechanism for its activation within the School of Dentistry.

Planning and Training

Each department is obligated to have its faculty maintain certification in CPR and to formulate its specific medical emergency plan and, if necessary, to activate the Medical Emergency Protocol formulated by the Oral and Maxillofacial Surgery Department, Medical College of Georgia, School of Dentistry. Compliance with the development of Departmental Medical Emergency plans will be monitored by the Oral and Maxillofacial Surgery Department.

It is the responsibility of the faculty/practitioner to provide initial management of the patient until the medical emergency response team arrives. Therefore, it is recommended that each department have frequent scheduled and unscheduled medical emergencies practice sessions, as part of the medical emergency plan.

Scheduled and unscheduled medical emergencies practice sessions will be part of the School of Dentistry's Medical Emergency Protocol throughout the school.

Medical Emergency Response Team

The designated medical emergency response team in the School of Dentistry will carry pagers that are keyed to the MCG medical emergency operator.

The designated response team includes: Oral Surgery faculty, residents and nurses.

1. MEDICAL EMERGENCY PROCEDURES

   During any MEDICAL EMERGENCY when assistance is needed call the MCG emergency operator (1-2222) and request activation of CODE *#66*.

   The activation of Code #66 will alert all members of the dental school emergency response team as to the location of the medical emergency in the dental school. Every individual on the response team who is on campus will respond to the emergency. Exceptions to the policy will be those critical individuals that are actively involved with patient treatment in the operating room or sedated patients in the clinic.

The medical emergency response team at the School of Dentistry will respond as noted above with the activation of Code #66.

Upon activation of Code #66 the members of response team that are physically on campus will respond to the emergency situation except for those critical personnel involved with patient care as noted above.

A designated code #66 flow-sheet will be filled out for each emergency situation. At a minimum the information listed below should be included on all flow-sheet.

— Time emergency recognized
— Time resuscitation begun
— Time telephone calls made
— Time any drugs administered and which ones
— Time help arrived
— Time patient recovered or was moved to hospital
— Time of any other pertinent actions
— Drs. attending

After initial assessment, a decision will be made by the emergency response team as to the disposition of the patient.

Emergency

1. Call 1-2222
2. Tell the operator to "Activate CODE #66 for a patient located in the School of Dentistry, Floor, Clinic # ."

3. Send individuals to the elevator and stairway to meet the response team to direct them to the emergency.
4. Send someone else to retrieve the emergency cart located in .

Note: If no response within five minutes, reactivate the initial Code and call 911.

Dental Emergency Care Policies and Procedures

A. Emergency Care for Assigned Patients

1. The provider is responsible for the complete oral health care of his/her assigned patients including emergency treatment. Providers should give each assigned patient his/her phone number and instruct the patient to contact him/her first if an emergency situation arises.
2. When contacted by a patient in need of emergency care, the student/provider should arrange to see the patient in a timely manner in the appropriate departmental clinic if possible. If the student/provider's schedule does not permit this, the student may arrange for his/her patient to be seen in the Emergency Dental Service (EDS).
3. To arrange for care in the EDS, the student/provider should contact Admissions (721-2371). Scheduling of patients, obtaining charts, and all administrative processing prior to being seen is accomplished by Admissions personnel. Patients should not be told to report to Admissions for emergency treatment without prior arrangement by the student dentist.

B. Normal Operations of the Emergency Dental Service

1. The Emergency Dental Service is available to all adults (age 14 or older) who request urgent dental

care including those with no previous care at MCG School of Dentistry.

2. The goal of the Emergency Dental Service is to treat urgent dental problems and to provide palliative relief for symptomatic conditions in an expeditious manner.
3. Normal hours of operation for the EDS are Monday - Friday from 12:30 - 5:00 PM. The clinic is closed during student breaks, exam week and other periods when students are unavailable for clinic assignment.

Emergency Care When School is Not in Session

Dental emergencies may be treated in the school only during normal clinic hours when the school is open. Evening and weekends and days when the school is closed, emergency patients may be seen in the hospital ER only.

Evenings/Weekends: The patient should first call his assigned student who will call 721-3893 (Paging and Locator Service) and ask the operator to page the General Practice Resident on call. If necessary, the student will meet the patient at the MCG Hospital Emergency Room and the resident will supervise the emergency treatment or suggest appropriate consultation. Should it be impossible for the patient to contact the student after normal school hours, the patient should have been advised earlier by the student to call 721-3893 (MCG Emergency Services) and ask the operator to page the resident on call. Emergency treatment will be accomplished in the Medical College of Georgia Hospital. Patients will be billed by the Medical College of Georgia Hospital for these services.

Holidays, Breaks and Periods When Students are Not Available in EDS.

Patients of record experiencing emergency dental

problems should contact the Patient Admissions Office at (706) 721-2371 and schedule an appointment for emergency treatment. The patient will be triaged by faculty and taken to the appropriate department for treatment.

Emergency Supervision for Patients with Acute Periodontal Problems

The dentist or dental student providing treatment for any patient will be responsible for the treatment of any emergency problem that may arise. For those emergencies which occur after school hours, the general policies and procedures for providing this treatment are listed below.

(a) Dental Students. Dental Students will contact the Periodontics Resident concerning the emergency problem. Contact can be obtained by calling the page number (723-1150) and leaving a message for the resident. If the emergency is the result of periodontal surgery, during normal business hours, the dental student will contact the faculty member who was present during the treatment to evaluate the patient's problem. If the faculty member cannot be contacted, the student will page the Periodontic Resident by calling 723-1150 and leaving a message for the resident. The patients will be examined and treated in Clinic 11 of the School of Dentistry by the Periodontic resident or faculty. If the emergency occurs after hours or on weekends, the patient must be treated in the hospital emergency room.

(b) Faculty members or Periodontic residents. If the faculty members or Periodontic residents who are responsible for the treatment of a patient with an acute periodontal emergency cannot be contacted by the patient, then the patient should contact the Periodontic resident on call, again by calling (723-1150) and leaving a message.

Reporting Accidental Injuries. (Contact Mr. Michael Budd, Admissions)

(a) Should a patient accident/injury occur (related to dental therapy) the student should first report to the attending faculty member.

IF THE ACCIDENT IS LIFE THREATENING, follow the Medical Emergency Protocol for the School of Dentistry.

If the accident/injury is NOT life threatening, the student and patient should report to Admissions to fill out an "Employee's Report of Accident/Injury" form. Detailed instructions for completing this form and follow-up activity (Emergency Room, blood testing, etc.) are available in Admissions.

If the accident/injury is NOT related to dental therapy, (patient falls, slips on wet floor, trips on stairs, etc.), the Admissions personnel will fill out the proper forms. If medical treatment is required, Public Safety will be called.

(a) Incident Reports

An incident is defined as adverse, unexpected occurrence of sufficient magnitude that it has the potential to be a risk management situation. Examples of instances for which incident reports are necessary include (1) required emergency medical attention by persons other than the attending dental staff for medical situations arising during the course of treatment, (2) injuries to the patient of significant magnitude that they require medical or surgical intervention, (3) dental treatment which is so substandard as to be judged grossly negligent, (4) any threat of legal action by any patient for treatment/diagnosis or the lack thereof, (5) death.

Reports should be filed by the attending dental staff and forwarded to the Chairperson, Quality Assurance Committee, MCG School of Dentistry within 24 hours. Information required is listed below:

- Name of patient
- Patient number or identifier
- Date of occurrence
- Location of patient at time of occurrence
- Individual reporting
- Date of report
- Brief summary, i.e. anaphylactic reaction, angina, threat of legal action
- Detailed description of event (copies of treatment report, if completed in detail, may suffice)

Reporting Needle Sticks, Cuts, and Treatment Related Injuries

1. All needle sticks and sharp instrument cuts inflicted on students must be reported immediately to their supervising faculty member. Exposures considered significant* include:
2. Needle sticks with contaminated needles
3. Puncture wounds from contaminated, sharp dental instruments
4. Contamination of any obviously open wound or the mucous membranes with saliva, blood, or a mixture of both saliva and blood
   - Exposure to a patient's blood or saliva on the unbroken skin is not considered significant.

Procedure for the Emergency Dental Service

Admissions (721-2371) is the initial entry point for the EDS and provide information and administrative support.

(a) For assigned patients, if their student cannot, for valid reasons, provide urgent care, the student should contact Admissions to arrange for treatment in the EDS.

(b) New patients can directly obtain information on clinic hours, fees and request treatment from Admissions. Patients are seen on a first-come, first-served basis. "Fee Tickets" are sequenced numerically to identify those who present earliest.

(c) For Assigned Patients, existing dental records are used to record all treatment. For new patients, an emergency record consisting of a record jacket, health history, treatment record, radiographic exposure log, and registration form is constructed

Protocol for Injury Management

1. Immediately cleanse the wound thoroughly with soap and water

2. The patient and the dental health care provider (student or assistant or faculty member involved) report to Mr. Michael Budd - Dental Admissions - for further instructions (as discussed in section 2.5).

3. Obtain the patient's and exposure recipient's permission for blood testing and arrange for pretest counseling.

4. Hepatitis Blood Test Results and Treatment Recommendations

A. HBsAg Negative (PATIENT)

   1. Hepatitis vaccine if not already received (STUDENT)

B. HBsAg Positive (PATIENT)

   1. If recipient is already anti-HBsAg positive: No treatment (STUDENT).

2. If recipient has had Hepatitis B vaccine with laboratory proven seroconversion: No treatment (STUDENT)
3. If recipient has had Hepatitis B vaccine without laboratory proven seroconversion: One additional dose of vaccine and one dose of HBIG if anti-HBs negative on testing. (STUDENT)
4. If recipient is negative for anti-HBs:
   — Start HBIG within 48 hours of exposure (0.06 ml/kg IM) and hepatitis B vaccination series within 7 days. (STUDENT)
   — HIV Blood Test Results and Treatment Recommendations

C. Diagnosed AIDS, anti-HIV (+), refuses testing or unknown source (PATIENT)
   1. If recipient is anti-HIV (+): should receive post-test counseling and medical evaluation (STUDENT)
   2. If recipient is anti-HIV (-): should receive post-test counseling and repeat testing at 6, 12, and 24 weeks. (STUDENT)

D. Anti-HIV (-) (PATIENT)
   1. If recipient is anti-HIV (+): should receive post-test counseling and medical evaluation (STUDENT).
   2. If recipient is anti-HIV (-): should receive post-test counseling and optional follow-up at 12 weeks. (STUDENT).

PROPERTY CODE: HOSPITAL AND EMERGENCY MEDICAL SERVICES LIENS

In this study:

1. "Emergency medical services" has the meaning assigned by Section 773.003, Health and Safety Code.
2. "Emergency medical services provider" has the meaning assigned by Section 773.003, Health and Safety Code.
3. "Hospital" means a person or institution maintaining a facility that provides hospital services in this state.
4. "Person" does not include a county, common, or independent school district.

Acts 1983, 68th Leg., p. 3562, ch. 576, — 1, eff. Jan. 1, 1984. Amended by Acts 2003, 78th Leg., ch. 337, — 1, eff. Sept. 1, 2003.

55.002. Lien

(a) A hospital has a lien on a cause of action or claim of an individual who receives hospital services for injuries caused by an accident that is attributed to the negligence of another person. For the lien to attach, the individual must be admitted to a hospital not later than 72 hours after the accident.

(b) The lien extends to both the admitting hospital and a hospital to which the individual is transferred for treatment of the same injury.

(c) An emergency medical services provider has a lien on a cause of action or claim of an individual who receives emergency medical services in a county with a population of 575,000 or less for injuries caused by an accident that is attributed to the negligence of another person. For the lien to attach, the individual must receive the emergency medical services not later than 72 hours after the accident.

Acts 1983, 68th Leg., p. 3562, ch. 576, — 1, eff. Jan. 1, 1984. Amended by Acts 2003, 78th Leg., ch. 337, — 1, eff. Sept. 1, 2003.

55.003. Property to Which Lien Attaches

(a) A lien under this chapter attaches to:

1. a cause of action for damages arising from an injury for which the injured individual is admitted to the hospital or receives emergency medical services;
2. a judgment of a court in this state or the decision of a public agency in a proceeding brought by the injured individual or by another person entitled to bring the suit in case of the death of the individual to recover damages arising from an injury for which the injured individual is admitted to the hospital or receives emergency medical services; and
3. the proceeds of a settlement of a cause of action or a claim by the injured individual or another person entitled to make the claim, arising from an injury for which the injured individual is admitted to the hospital or receives emergency medical services.

(b) The lien does not attach to:

1. a claim under the workers' compensation law of this state, the Federal Employees Liability Act, or the Federal Longshore and Harbor Workers' Compensation Act; or
2. the proceeds of an insurance policy in favour of the injured individual or the injured individual's beneficiary or legal representative, except public liability insurance carried by the insured that protects the insured against loss caused by an accident or collision.

(c) A hospital lien described by Section 55.002(a) does not attach to a claim against the owner or operator of a railroad company that maintains or whose employees maintain a hospital in which the injured individual is receiving hospital services.

Acts 1983, 68th Leg., p. 3562, ch. 576, § 1, eff. Jan. 1, 1984. Amended by Acts 2003, 78th Leg., ch. 337, § 1, eff. Sept. 1, 2003.

55.004. Amount of Lien

(a) In this section, "emergency hospital care" means health care services provided in a hospital to evaluate, stabilize, and treat a serious medical problem of recent onset or severity, including severe pain that would lead a prudent layperson possessing an average knowledge of medicine and health to believe that the condition, illness, or injury is of such a nature that failure to obtain immediate medical care would in all reasonable probability:

1. seriously jeopardize the patient's health;
2. seriously impair one or more bodily functions;
3. seriously harm an organ or other part of the body;
4. cause serious disfigurement; or
5. in the case of a pregnant woman, seriously jeopardize the health of the fetus.

(b) A hospital lien described by Section 55.002(a) is for the amount of the hospital's charges for services provided to the injured individual during the first 100 days of the injured individual's hospitalisation.

(c) A hospital lien described by Section 55.002(a) may also include the amount of a physician's reasonable and necessary charges for emergency hospital care services provided to the injured individual during the first seven days of the injured individual's hospitalisation. At the request of the physician, the hospital may act on the physician's behalf in securing and discharging the lien.

(d) A hospital lien described by Section 55.002(a) does not cover:

1. charges for other services that exceed a reasonable and regular rate for the services;
2. charges by the physician related to any services provided under Subsection (c) for which the physician has accepted insurance benefits or payment under a private medical indemnity plan or program, regardless of whether the benefits or payment equals the full amount of the physician's charges for those services;
3. charges by the physician for services provided under Subsection (c) if the injured individual has coverage under a private medical indemnity plan or program from which the physician is entitled to recover payment for the physician's services under an assignment of benefits or similar rights; or
4. charges by the physician related to any services provided under Subsection (c) if the physician is a member of the legislature.

(e) A hospital lien described by Section 55.002(a) is not affected by a hospital's use of a method of classifying patients according to their ability to pay that is solely intended to obtain a lien for services provided to an indigent injured individual.

(f) An emergency medical services lien described by Section 55.002(c) is for the amount charged by the emergency medical services provider, not to exceed $1,000, for emergency medical services provided to the injured individual during the 72 hours following the accident that caused the individual's injuries.

(g) An emergency medical services lien described by Section 55.002(c) does not cover:

1. charges for services that exceed a reasonable and regular rate for the services;
2. charges by the emergency medical services provider related to any services for which the emergency medical services provider has accepted insurance benefits or payment under a private medical indemnity plan or program, regardless of whether the benefits or payments equal the full amount of the charges for those services; or
3. charges by the emergency medical services provider for services provided if the injured individual has coverage under a private medical indemnity plan or program from which the provider is entitled to recover payment for the provider's services under an assignment of benefits or similar right.

(h) If the physician is employed in that capacity by an institution of higher education, as defined by Section 61.003, Education Code, and the lien does not include the amount of the physician's reasonable and necessary charges described by Subsection (c), the physician has a lien on the cause of action in the same manner as a hospital under this chapter. The lien is subject to provisions of this chapter applicable to a hospital lien, and the physician or the physician's employing institution may secure and enforce the lien in the manner provided by this chapter.

Acts 1983, 68th Leg., p. 3563, ch. 576, § 1, eff. Jan. 1, 1984. Amended by Acts 2001, 77th Leg., ch. 930, § 1, eff. Sept. 1, 2001; Acts 2003, 78th Leg., ch. 337, § 1, eff. Sept.

1, 2003; Acts 2003, 78th Leg., ch. 1266, § 1.16, eff. June 20, 2003; Acts 2005, 79th Leg., ch. 728, § 23.001(79), eff. Sept. 1, 2005.

55.005. Securing Lien

(a) To secure the lien, a hospital or emergency medical services provider must file written notice of the lien with the county clerk of the county in which the services were provided. The notice must be filed before money is paid to an entitled person because of the injury.

(b) The notice must contain:

1. the injured individual's name and address;
2. the date of the accident;
3. the name and location of the hospital or emergency medical services provider claiming the lien; and
4. the name of the person alleged to be liable for damages arising from the injury, if known.

(c) The county clerk shall record the name of the injured individual, the date of the accident, and the name and address of the hospital or emergency medical services provider and shall index the record in the name of the injured individual.

Acts 1983, 68th Leg., p. 3563, ch. 576, * 1, eff. Jan. 1, 1984. Amended by Acts 1995, 74th Leg., ch. 1031, * 1, eff. Aug. 28, 1995; Acts 2003, 78th Leg., ch. 337, * 1, eff. Sept. 1, 2003.

55.006. Discharge of Lien

(a) To discharge a lien under this chapter, the authorities of the hospital or emergency medical services provider claiming the lien or the person in charge of the finances of the hospital or emergency medical services provider must execute and file with the county clerk of the county in which the lien notice was filed a certificate stating that the debt covered by the lien has been paid or released and authorizing the clerk to discharge the lien.

(b) The county clerk shall record a memorandum of the certificate and the date it was filed.

(c) The filing of the certificate and recording of the memorandum discharge the lien.

Acts 1983, 68th Leg., p. 3564, ch. 576, * 1, eff. Jan. 1, 1984. Amended by Acts 2003, 78th Leg., ch. 337, * 1, eff. Sept. 1, 2003.

55.007. Validity of Release

(a) A release of a cause of action or judgment to which a lien under this chapter may attach is not valid unless:

1. the charges of the hospital or emergency medical services provider claiming the lien were paid in full before the execution and delivery of the release;
2. the charges of the hospital or emergency medical services provider claiming the lien were paid before the execution and delivery of the release to the extent of any full and true consideration paid to the injured individual by or on behalf of the other parties to the release; or
3. the hospital or emergency medical services provider claiming the lien is a party to the release.

(b) A judgment to which a lien under this chapter has attached remains in effect until the charges of the hospital or emergency medical services provider claiming the lien are paid in full or to the extent set out in the judgment.

Acts 1983, 68th Leg., p. 3564, ch. 576, * 1, eff. Jan. 1,

1984. Amended by Acts 2003, 78th Leg., ch. 337, * 1, eff. Sept. 1, 2003.

55.008. Records

(a) On request by an attorney for a party by, for, or against whom a claim is asserted for damages arising from an injury, a hospital or emergency medical services provider shall as promptly as possible make available for the attorney's examination its records concerning the services provided to the injured individual.

(b) The hospital or emergency medical services provider may issue reasonable rules for granting access to its records under this section, but it may not deny access because a record is incomplete.

(c) The records are admissible, subject to applicable rules of evidence, in a civil suit arising from the injury.

Acts 1983, 68th Leg., p. 3564, ch. 576, * 1, eff. Jan. 1, 1984. Amended by Acts 2003, 78th Leg., ch. 337, * 1, eff. Sept. 1, 2003.

HEART ATTACK TREATMENTS

Most communities have an emergency cardiovascular care system that can respond quickly. This prompt care dramatically reduces heart damage. In fact, 88 percent of heart attack survivors under age 65 can return to their usual work. Prompt care isn't the only reason so many heart attack survivors recover so quickly, but it's an important one.

If a victim gets to an emergency room fast enough, reperfusion (rep"er-FU'zhun) therapy may be done. This increases blood supply to the heart muscle. It's done with drugs to dissolve clots (thrombolysis), balloon angioplasty

(PTCA) or surgery. The sooner any of these techniques occur, the more likely the patient will benefit.

Thrombolysis (throm"bo-LI'sis) involves injecting a clot-dissolving agent, such as streptokinase, urokinase or tPA (tissue plasminogen activator), to dissolve a clot in a coronary artery and restore blood flow. For best effect, these drugs must be used within a few (usually 3) hours of a heart attack.

If this treatment isn't done immediately after a heart attack, percutaneous transluminal coronary angioplasty (per"ku-TA'ne-us tranz-LU'min-al KOR'o-nair-e AN'je-o-plas-te) (PTCA) or coronary artery bypass graft surgery (CABG) may be done later to improve blood supply to the heart muscle. Once part of the heart muscle dies, its function can't be restored. However, function may be restored to areas with decreased blood flow.

AHA Recommendation

When a heart attack occurs, you must recognize the signals and respond immediately. Time is critical. When an artery to the heart (coronary artery) is blocked, the heart muscle doesn't die instantly. But damage increases the longer the artery stays blocked. Delay may increase heart damage and reduce your chance of survival. It also lessens the chance of preserving heart muscle. This increases the risk of disability.

Anyone who has heart attack warning signs should call 9-1-1 immediately. People who pass out before reaching the emergency room should receive cardiopulmonary resuscitation (kar"de-o-PUL'mo-nair-e re-sus"ah-TA'shun) (CPR).

Related AHA Publications

— Heart and Stroke Facts

- After Your Heart Attack (also in Spanish)
- Aspirin and Your Health
- About Your Bypass Surgery
- Your Cardiac Catheterisation and Coronary Arteriography
- Your PTCA
- "What Is Coronary Angioplasty?", "What Is Coronary Bypass Surgery?", "What Is Echocardiography?", "How Will I Recover From My Heart Attack?" and "What Is Cardiac Rehabilitation?" in Answers By Heart kit

"CLOSED" INTENSIVE CARE UNITS AND OTHER MODELS OF CARE FOR CRITICALLY ILL PATIENTS

Patients in the intensive care unit (ICU) require complex care relating to a broad range of acute illnesses and pre-existing conditions. The innate complexity of the ICU makes organisational structuring of care an attractive quality measure and a target for performance improvement strategies. In other words, organisational features relating to medical and nursing leadership, communication and collaboration among providers, and approaches to problem-solving may capture the quality of ICU care more comprehensively than do practices related to specific processes of care.

Most features of ICU organisation do not exert a demonstrable impact on clinical outcomes such as morbidity and mortality. While hard clinical outcomes may not represent the most appropriate measure of success for many organisational features, the role of "intensivists" (specialists in critical care medicine) in managing ICU patients has shown a beneficial impact on patient outcomes in a number of studies. For this reason, the Leapfrog Group, representing

Fortune 500 corporations and other large healthcare purchasers, has identified staffing ICUs with intensivists as one of three recommended hospital safety initiatives for its 2000 purchasing principles.

In this chapter, we review the benefits of full-time intensivists and the impact of "closed ICUs" (defined below) on patient outcomes. Much of this literature makes no distinction between improved outcomes in general and decreased harm in particular. However, given the high mortality and complication rates observed in ICUs, it seems reasonable to consider global interventions such as organisational changes as patient safety practices.

Practice Description

The following practice definitions are synthesized from studies reviewed for this chapter. For all of these models, the term "intensivist" refers to a physician with primary training in medicine, surgery, anesthesiology or pediatrics followed by 2-3 years of critical care medicine (CCM) training.

Intensivist Co-management—An open ICU model in which all patients receive mandatory consultation from an intensivist. The internist, family physician, or surgeon remains a co-attending-of-record with intensivists collaborating in the management of all ICU patients.

Closed ICU model—An ICU in which patients admitted to the ICU are transferred to the care of an intensivist assigned to the ICU on a full-time basis. Generally, patients are accepted to the ICU only after approval/evaluation by the intensivist. For periods typically ranging from one week to one month at a time, the intensivist's clinical duties predominantly consist of caring for patients in the ICU, with no concurrent outpatient responsibilities.

Open ICU model—An ICU in which patients are admitted

under the care of an internist, family physician, surgeon or other primary attending of record, with intensivists available providing expertise via elective consultation. Intensivists may play a *de facto* primary role in the management of some patients, but only within the discretion of the attending-of-record.

Open ICU model—An ICU in which patients are admitted under the care of an internist, family physician, surgeon or other primary attending of record, with intensivists available providing expertise via elective consultation. Intensivists may play a *de facto* primary role in the management of some patients, but only within the discretion of the attending-of-record.

Mixed ICU models—In practice, the above models overlap to a considerable extent. Thus, some studies avoid attempting to characterize ICUs in terms of these models and focus instead on the level of involvement of intensivists in patient care regardless of the organisational model. This involvement may consist of daily ICU rounds by an intensivist (thus including "closed model ICUs" and "intensivist comanagement"), ICU directorship by an intensivist (possibly including examples of all 3 models above), or simply the presence of a full-time intensivist in the ICU (also including examples of all 3 models.)

Intensivist models—ICU management may include all of these models. These models are contrasted with the open ICU model, in which an intensivist generally does not participate in the direct care of a significant proportion of the ICU patients.

Prevalence and Severity of the Target Safety Problem

ICUs comprise approximately 10% of acute care hospital beds. The number of annual ICU admissions in the United

State is estimated to be 4.4 million patients. Due to an aging population and the increasing acuity of illness of hospitalized patients, both the total number of ICU patients and their proportional share of hospital admissions overall are expected to grow.

ICU patients have, on average, mortality rates between 12 and 17%. Overall, approximately 500,000 ICU patients die annually in the United States. A recent review estimated that this mortality could be reduced by 15 to 60% using an intensivist model of ICU management.

Young and Birkmeyer have provided estimates of the relative reduction in annual ICU mortalities resulting from conversion of all urban ICUs to an intensivist model of management model. Using conservative estimates for current ICU mortality rates of 12%, and estimating that 85% of urban ICUs are not currently intensivist-managed, the authors calculated that approximately 360,000 patients die annually in urban ICUs without intensivists. A conservative projection of a 15% relative reduction in mortality resulting from intensivist-managed ICUs yields a predicted annual saving of nearly 54,000 lives.

By only measuring ICU mortality rates, this analysis may underestimate the importance of intensivist-managed ICUs. In addition to mortality, other quality of care outcome measures that might be improved by intensivists include rates of ICU complications, inappropriate ICU utilisation, patient suffering, appropriate end-of-life palliative care, and futile care.

Study Designs

Among 14 studies abstracted for this chapter, 2 were systematic reviews and 12 were original studies. One systematic review is an abstract that has not yet appeared in journal form and does not provide cited references. The other systematic review evaluated 8 references, all of which are included in this chapter. An additional 4 studies absent from the systematic review are included here. These 4 studies include 2 abstracts that were published after the 1999 systematic review, and 2 studies of pediatric ICUs with intensivists.

Among the original studies, 6 incorporated historical controls and 5 used a cross-sectional approach. One study had both historical and cross-sectional components. The original studies include 4 studies of adult medical ICUs, 6 studies of adult surgical ICUs and 2 studies of pediatric multidisciplinary ICUs. Intensivist models used by the studies cited for this review include 4 closed ICUs, 4 mixed ICUs, 3 ICUs with intensivist comanagement and one open ICU.

Several studies were excluded, including abstracts with insufficient data, unclear distinctions in patient management between control groups and intervention (intensivist managed) groups, intensivist models that may have important roles in future practice (e.g., telemedicine consultation with remote management) but are not yet widely available and considerably older studies.

Opportunities for Impact

Currently, a minority of ICUs in the United States utilizes the intensivist model of ICU management. Intensivists are even less frequently found in non-teaching and rural hospitals. The potential impact of the intensivist model is far-reaching.

Evidence for Effectiveness of the Practice

Most of the studies report a decrease in unadjusted in-hospital mortality and/or ICU mortality, although this decrease did not reach statistical significance in 3 of the 14 studies. One study found a statistically insignificant increase in the unadjusted mortality rates associated with the intensivist model ICU. This study also found that the ratio of expected-to-actual mortality was reduced in the intensivist-model ICUs. This finding was associated with a higher severity of illness scores in the intensivist-model ICU population. A similar finding of significantly improved outcomes after adjusting for severity of illness and comparing expected-to-actual mortality rates was demonstrated in one pediatric study. Overall, the relative risk reduction for ICU mortality ranges from 29% to 58%. The relative risk reduction for overall hospital mortality is 23% to 50%. These results are consistent with those of a previous systematic review that found a 15% to 65% reduction in mortality rates in intensivist-managed ICUs.

Data concerning long-term survival (6 and 12 months) for patients cared for in ICUs with and without intensivist management is not available. Differences in outcomes between closed ICUs, mixed ICU models and co-managed ICUs are difficult to assess. Studies that have addressed conversion from an open to a closed model did not utilize full-time intensivists in the open model study phases. Therefore it is not clear to what extent improved patient outcomes resulted only from changes in intensivists' direct patient care and supervision.

The observational studies evaluating these practices suffer from 2 major limitations. Half of the studies retrospectively compared post-implementation outcomes with those during an historical control period. Because none of these studies included a similar comparison for a control unit that remained open in both time periods, we lack information on secular trends in ICU outcomes during the time periods evaluated. The other major limitation associated with comparing mortality rates for ICU patients relates to differences in ICU admission and discharge criteria under different organisational models. Under the intensivist model, patients are generally accepted to the ICU only after approval/ evaluation by the intensivist. Thus, conversion to an intensivist model ICU may bring about changes in the ICU patient population that are incompletely captured by risk-adjustment models and confound comparisons of mortality rates. Moreover, these changes in ICU admitting practice may exert contradictory effects. For example, an intensivist model ICU may result in fewer ICU admissions for patients with dismal prognoses, and less futile care for patients already in the ICU. On the other hand, intensivist-managed ICUs with stricter admission and discharge criteria may result in a greater overall acuity of illness for the ICU patients and therefore higher mortality rates.

Study Outcomes

Required outcomes of interest in studies chosen for this chapter were ICU mortality, overall in-hospital mortality, or both. Some studies also included morbidity outcomes, adverse events and resource utilisation (e.g., length of ICU and hospital stay), levels of patient acuity or severity of illness (ICU utilisation) and levels of high-intensity intervention usage. Studies addressing the impact of intensivist ICU management on resource utilisation without mortality or outcome data were excluded. There are no data regarding the impact of intensivists.

Costs and Implementation

These studies did not address the incremental costs associated with implementation of full-time intensivists. Several studies have analysed resource utilisation and length of stay associated with intensivist-managed ICUs. The results of these studies are variable with respect to costs. Some demonstrate a decrease in ICU expenses. Others found increased costs, likely due to the increased use of expensive technologies. Still others show little overall cost differential. The cost-effectiveness and cost-benefit of an intensivist-model ICU requires further study.

Comment

Outcomes research in critical care is particularly challenging for several reasons. It typically relies on observational outcomes studies, and must account for the diversity and complexity of variables measured and controlled for, such as patient-based, disease-based, provider-based and therapy-based variables. Despite these challenges and limitations, the literature fairly clearly shows that intensivists favourably impact ICU patient outcomes. What remains unclear is which intensivist model to recommend—intensivist consultation versus intensivist co-management versus closed ICUs. Also, we do not know the degree to which the choice among these models depends on intensivist background—i.e., medicine, anesthesiology or surgery. Finally, because the mechanism of the benefit of intensivist models is unknown, the degree to which this benefit can be captured by other changes in practice (e.g., adoption of certain evidence-based processes of ICU care) remains unclear.

The major incentive for clarifying these issues concerns the implications for staffing ICUs in the future. While the evidence supports the beneficial role of full-time intensivists, the current number of trainees is insufficient to keep pace with the expected increase in the number of ICU patients. Until we are able to sufficiently increase the size and number of CCM training programs for physician specialists, complementary solutions for meeting critical care management demands should be considered. These might include incorporating physician-extenders such as nurse practitioners and physician assistants with specialized critical care training, increased participation by hospitalists in care of ICU patients, regionalisation of critical care services, or providing innovative methods to extend intensivists' expertise to remote sites through telemedicine consultations. The latter practice seems particularly promising—a recent time series cohort study found an approximately 33% decrease in severity-adjusted hospital mortality and a nearly 50% decrease in ICU complications when a technology-enabled remote ICU management program was instituted in a community-based ICU.

Potential for Harm

The potential for harm resulting from intensivist management is unclear. Concerns raised in the literature about intensivist-managed ICUs include the loss of continuity of care by primary care physicians, insufficient patient-specific knowledge by the intensivist, reduced use of necessary sub-specialist consultations, and inadequate CCM training of residents who formerly managed their own ICU patients. Perhaps more worrisome is the impact that adoption of this practice would have on physician staffing and workforce requirements. Without a substantial increase in the numbers of physicians trained in CCM, projected increases in the ICU patient population over the next 30 years will result in a significant shortfall in the intensivist workforce.

RHEUMATOLOGIC TECHNICAL PROCEDURES

The Starred Surgical Procedures

In addition to the major global surgeries in the Surgery section of the AMA CPT, manual, there are a number of minor surgeries designated by a star (*) following the procedure code. These starred minor surgeries involve a readily identifiable surgical procedure but include variable preoperative and postoperative services (e.g., injection of a tendon sheath and manipulation of a joint under anesthesia). Because of the indefinite preoperative and postoperative services, they are not traditionally paid using a global surgery policy.

The star indicates that the usual preoperative and postoperative period of 30 days for major global surgeries does not apply. Most minor surgeries performed by rheumatologists have no postoperative period. There are no postoperative periods for arthrocentesis (20600*, 20605*, and 20610*), a needle muscle biopsy (20206*), and an injection of a tender sheath or trigger point (20550*). Because the 10-day postoperative period was eliminated for 20550*, CPT modifiers "-24" and "-79" should no longer be used with this code. If a minor surgery with no postoperative period and an unrelated office service are provided, then CPT modifier "-25," "significant, separately identifiable evaluation and management service by the same physician on the same day of a procedure or other service," should be used. This circumstance should be reported by adding the modifier "-25" to the E/M service code (or indicated by 09925) in addition to coding for the procedure. *HCFA does not recognize starred procedures. The procedures eligible for a "-25" modifier are those with zero or 10 post-operative days. Those with a 90-day global period are not.* In the past, some Medicare carriers have requested two ICD-9-CM codes, one for the E/M service and one for the procedure. While carriers have been instructed not to request two diagnosis codes in this situation, it is advisable to check with your carrier to determine their preferences. Keep in mind that carriers may also require additional documentation from rheumatologists whose utilisation significantly exceeds the norm.

In the alphanumeric section of HCPCS, there are separate "J" codes available to report the drug costs for joint or soft tissue injections as well as gold or methotrexate injections (i.e., J9260 methotrexate 50 mg.). Payment for drugs by Medicare is based on 95 percent of the average wholesale price. Administration of injections, such as gold, methotrexate, ACTH, depo-steroid IM and Colchicine (CPT 90782-90788) will only be reimbursed by Medicare when not provided in conjunction with an E/M service or procedure. Therefore, there are two methods to report these injections: (1) if provided on the same day as an E/M service, code for the office visit and the drug cost, or (2) if not provided on the same day, code for the administration of the injection and the drug cost.

Some examples of rheumatologic technical procedures which are not starred minor surgeries and therefore cannot be accompanied by an E/M service code include: CPT code 42405, (an incisional biopsy of the salivary gland), CPT code 40490 (a lip biopsy), CPT code 11100 (a biopsy of the skin), or CPT code 20205 (a deep muscle biopsy).

Rheumatologists may also commonly perform perineural injections, for example, for patients with carpal tunnel syndrome. Use CPT code 20550 to indicate this procedure.

Certain procedures are a combination of a physician professional component and a technical component. When the physician component is reported separately, the service may be identified by adding the modifier "-26" to the usual procedure code (or indicated by 09926). For example, if bilateral x-rays of the wrist are ordered for a patient who has the procedure done in the radiology department of a community hospital, it would be coded as 73100-26 twice (73100-26 RT and 73100-26 LT) to indicate bilateral radiologic examination of the wrist, anteroposterior and lateral views, physician component. You can also code 73100 once and put a "2" in the units column of the claim form. Most carriers prefer that the above example be coded as 73100-26-50 (the payment modifier should always be listed first). Some carriers may prefer that the above example be coded as 73100-99, 09950, 09926. All carriers are working towards a universal reporting system that will ensure national standards. Check with your carrier to determine its local policy.

CPT codes for diagnostic and interventional arthroscopy of many joints, as well as synovectomy by arthroscopy can be found in the arthroscopy section of the AMA CPT manual (CPT 29800 through 29909). As outlined in the manual, surgical arthroscopy always includes a diagnostic arthroscopy. When an arthroscopy is performed in conjunction with an arthrotomy, the modifier "-51" should be added to the secondary procedure (or indicated by 09951) which alerts the carrier that "multiple procedures" were performed. HCFA will pay the lesser of the actual charge or 100 percent of the fee schedule amount for the most expensive procedure. Payment for the second through fifth procedure will be based on the lesser of the actual charge or 50 percent of the fee schedule amount. Each procedure after the fifth procedure will require additional documentation before payment is made. *Note: It may be useful to know that your Medicare carrier will automatically apply modifier "-51" when multiple procedures are billed on the same day. Use of this modifier then becomes less important from a payment standpoint and other payment modifiers should be listed first.*

If a bilateral procedure is performed, the modifier "-50" or 09950 should be used. For example, if an arthrocentesis is performed on both knees, CPT code 20610-50 would be reported. Some carriers, however, prefer that the first arthrocentesis be coded as 20610 and the second (bilateral) arthrocentesis as 20610-50. You can also code 20610 once and put a "2" in the units column of the claim form. Check with your carrier to determine its local policy.

A service or procedure may be provided that is not listed in the AMA CPT manual. For this reason, "unlisted procedure" codes are available to indicate the service. Refer to the "Surgery Guidelines" section for additional information about coding for technical rheumatologic procedures. A complete description of the service provided, preferably an operative report, should accompany the claim form.

Rheumatologists who furnish any covered durable medical equipment, prosthetics, orthotics, supplies and other selected items (DMEPOS) to their patients are considered "suppliers." Rheumatologists will have to bill for the supplies separately to one of four regional carriers designated to handle claims for supplies. These regulations do not apply to rheumatologists who prescribe but do not supply and bill DMEPOS to their patients.

ST JOSEPH'S HOSPITAL, LONGFORD, THE REPUBLIC OF IRELAND

St Joseph's Hospital is a long-term residential and day care hospital for the elderly. The hospital had a change of management three years ago and will be joined by a new Director of Nursing in March 2002. Work Positive provided a morale boost for the staff as well as the opportunity for consultation, assisted senior management recognition of the changes needed within the hospital, therefore facilitating the implementation of these changes.

Step 1

Gaining Commitment

Work Positive was coordinated by the Health Promotion Specialist and the Director of Nursing. Two meetings were held with heads of departments and the Health and Safety Committee.

Demonstrating Commitment

The Director of Nursing supported the process from the beginning. In addition, feedback was provided to the wider health board.

Raising Awareness

A Health Promotion Specialist, from the Health Promotion Service, Midland Health Board, ran awareness sessions within focus groups. A one-page sheet detailing Work Positive was issued to each member of staff within these sessions.

Look at the Hazards and Benchmarking

Management staff independently completed the benchmark and discussed their responses. In addition, the Health Promotion Specialist facilitated a benchmark exercise, with a group of non-management staff. Thus, providing two perspectives for comparison.

Step 2

Decide Who Might be Harmed and How

164 employees were targeted at the hospital.

Step 3

Evaluate the Risks and Take Action Risk Assessment

Photocopies of the risk assessment questionnaire were issued to all staff via internal mail, along with a covering letter.

Forms were returned via a voting box in the main reception area. An initial response rate of 47% rose to 62% after a reminder memo had been issued.

Forms were analysed according to nine categories of

staff, using a statistical package to identify the proportion of responses per question.

Feedback to Staff

Copies of the analysis were made available to all staff. Results were also communicated via feedback sessions run by the Health Promotion Specialist, with high attendance from across the workforce.

Step 4

Developing Solutions

Solutions were discussed at the feedback sessions, with a mixed group of roles in each session. in each session.

A specialist in shift work was consulted.

Results

The Main Priority Issues

Within the hospital, priority issues appeared within one particular category of staff, i.e. the attendants, who have a dual role of domestic and caring duties.

- Shift work/patterns.
- Communication issues: feedback, follow-up of meetings, career appraisal, lack of consultation, involvement in decision-making.
- Workload: balancing domestic and caring duties.

Action Taken

- Consulted a specialist in shift work, who has met with attendants and managers and is currently producing two different rota proposals - which will then be voted on by the employees.
- Working day shortened and attendants are now paid for their morning break.

— Implementation of an appraisal system is being discussed with Human Resources and formalised programmes will be introduced in 2002.

— Further discussions are being held regarding the distribution of workload.

— Attendants are now involved in the morning team meeting. This aids communication and the breakdown of barriers between roles.

Lessons Learned

— An internal coordinator is needed to effectively facilitate the process.

— Analysis should be allocated to an appropriate person, due to the time involved.

2

General and Local Hospital Network Development

CRITICAL ACCESS HOSPITAL NETWORK DEVELOPMENT

Critical access hospitals (CAHs) are involved in a variety of networking relationships with local and regional health care providers and agencies. Organisational linkages range from very loose connections with little or no organisational commitment, to those that encompass a variety of local stakeholders organised to address mutually beneficial goals for their communities. The former tend to be based around meeting minimum programme standards while the latter tend to encompass more substantial areas of collaboration, while also involving a larger number of hospitals (and in some cases, non-hospital participants as well).

The vast majority of networking relationships meet minimum standards and little more. Network relationships that extend beyond the minimum standards are most common in those states that either incorporated additional standards into their state Flex Programme or had a pre-existing network development programme (e.g., North Dakota, Minnesota, Kansas, and Nebraska). States with prior network development initiatives incorporated the Flex Programme into their existing efforts rather than keeping it as a separate initiative. In some of these states (e.g., Michigan and North Carolina), the existing programmes provided a vehicle for involving CAH networks in a wide range of community-based programmes.

Given the historical market conditions that have faced many CAHs, it is not a surprise that only a few ventured beyond the minimum standards for participation. Observations of network development activities during the second year of the programme suggest a desire to move forward with hospital conversion as soon as possible.

External Linkages and Conversion/Post-Conversion Success

All but one of the CAHs in the survey reported having an affiliation agreement with another hospital. Since affiliation agreements are not all alike and relationships between CAHs and their affiliated hospitals can take a number of forms, some CAHs may be more or less prepared for conversion and post-conversion operations than others. In some cases the level of preparation for conversion could be due to the nature of the relationship with the affiliated hospital, while in others it could be due to prior affiliation experiences and the adaptive knowledge and/or momentum gained through such experiences.

Preparation for the operational requirements involved in becoming a CAH and the ability to avoid costly errors in organising for post-conversion operations can mean the difference between success and failure (i.e., leveraging pre-CAH network relationships to obtain capital and/or operational resources in an efficient and effective manner). Hospitals in the beginning stages of network development face a formidable learning curve (i.e., expending precious time, money and opportunities in their search for the best market fit). For example, one of the CAHs in the study had been exploring the benefits of outsourcing its laboratory services to a particular company. Upon discussion with a number of network members with experience in this area, the CAH decided it was not worth it. The insights gained during discussions with network partners were extracted from outsourcing experiences rather than feasibility analyses, and therefore were not otherwise available to the CAH.

One of the CAHs visited this year benefited from a strong affiliation with an urban tertiary care facility located about sixty miles away. Prior to conversion, the smaller rural hospital had operated at a significant loss (several hundred thousand dollars per year for a number of years). Its stronger network partner shouldered those losses, and only this year has taken a second look because of its own operational downturn. Converting to a CAH was an integral component in the network's strategy for stabilizing the smaller hospital.

In addition to the financial support provided, the support hospital also provided joint purchasing, administrative support (now provided through a management contract) and opportunities for continuing medical education for the CAH staff through its telemedicine system. The telemedicine system is also used for dermatology, wound care and radiology consultations. This network now includes twelve hospitals and has initiated efforts to coordinate peer review and quality improvement activities.

Why do support hospitals enter into the arrangements they do with CAHs? There are many possible reasons. The most obvious reason is self-interest. In some fashion organisational needs are being met for the support hospital (e.g., referrals, market protection, revenue stream from management fees). Although payment of management fees (i.e., contract management and/or other services contracts) is an explicit market transaction, CAHs can benefit immeasurably from their investments. In exchange for a management fee payment to its affiliated hospital, one CAH received recruitment support, management support, and group purchasing at an annual savings of approximately $250,000.

Another, less recognized reason involves more altruistic factors. Several cases were identified during our site visits where the support hospital was the anchor member of a network and had a distinct mission to assist local communities and their providers (i.e., benefit to the support hospital was not a prerequisite for support beyond allowing them to fulfill their mission statement). For others, it could stem from a particular point of view held by the support hospital's administrator and board. Often these types of network relationships were related to non-sectarian organisations, suggesting that mission may be a key influence. The subtlety of supportive relationships and their connection to effective versus minimal collaboration warrants further investigation in future work.

In addition to a unilateral mission effect, it also is possible that supportive linkages could be generated from more of a sense of shared purpose and mission (e.g., CAHs that are formal members of a provider system). In an effort to better understand these types of relationships, we divided the CAH sample into two groups: those in a linkage with a system or with a management contract, versus those that did not have these characteristics and were essentially freestanding institutions. We also explored differences between CAHs with pre-conversion affiliation agreements versus those hospitals that obtained such affiliations only after conversion to a CAH.

Forty-five percent of the CAHs in the sample were

identified as being owned or leased by a system or under a management contract (system), with the remaining hospitals identified as freestanding CAHs (freestanding). These two subgroups of CAHs exhibited slight differences in operating statistics. Freestanding CAHs had a slightly higher average number of set-up and staffed beds, slightly longer average length of stay for inpatients and slightly fewer medical professionals on staff. In terms of network linkages, the freestanding CAHs were more likely to link with freestanding support hospitals (i.e., 39% of system CAHs linked to freestanding facilities while nine in ten freestanding CAHs linked with freestanding hospitals).

A closer look at the freestanding and system affiliation agreements revealed that the two groups of hospitals prioritized major affiliation areas similarly. The top five areas for each group were identical, including rankings. These same five areas also demonstrated the greatest post-conversion change when compared to the others listed as major affiliation areas.

The sharing of these affiliation areas by freestanding and system facilities may reflect similar collective impressions of what is important to include in an affiliation agreement. Not surprisingly, the affiliation areas that increased the most were those areas most heavily stressed by the Flex Programme. Although the numbers are small, system CAHs were more likely than freestanding CAHs to have affiliation agreements for administrative support and specialty clinical personnel - networking features commonly associated with system membership.

Finally, the higher degree of involvement in non-medically related areas, such as administration support and financial support, for the system CAHs compared to the freestanding CAHs is consistent with system membership benefits and access to external resources and expertise through management contracts.

TABLE 1

Pre-Conversion Administrative Affiliation Areas by Hospital Linkage

	Freestanding CAHs (%)	*System Linked / Contract Managed CAHs (%)*
Administrative Support	39	75
Financial Support	22	63
Management Information System Support	18	53
Marketing/Public Relations Support	9	44

Table 2 provides a snapshot of the pre-conversion affiliation areas that are related to core hospital production areas (i.e., those areas most identified with the operational activities of the hospital). Benefits are apparent for the medical side as well as for hospitals with a system linkage or management contract.

TABLE 2

Pre-Conversion Operational Affiliation Areas by Hospital Linkage

	Freestanding CAHs (%)	*System Linked / Contract Managed CAHs (%)*
Specialty Clinic Support	59	79
Quality Related Support	42	60
Clinical Support	29	50
Primary Care Support	22	29

Availability of Health Care Services and CAH Linkages

Since the guidelines shaping the Flex Programme offer considerable flexibility for interpretation and implementation, it is not surprising that many participating hospitals report little if any operational change following conversion. It is also possible that the changes that have been reported could be the result of other unidentified actions that started prior to programme participation and which were complementary to conversion. The implications of prior network affiliation experiences and system or management contract linkage benefits were examined by dividing the sample of CAHs into four groups: 1) Freestanding CAHs that also had a pre-CAH linkage agreement with one or more providers; 2) Freestanding CAHs that did not have a pre-CAH agreement; 3) System Contract Managed CAHs that had a pre-CAH agreement; and 4) System Contract Managed CAHs that did not have a pre-CAH agreement. The last group represents facilities that either became linked with a system or formed a management contract at the time of conversion. These subgroups were then compared in terms of changes in scope of services following conversion. Post-conversion scope of service characteristics were defined as follows: 1) dropped as a service; 2) limited in scope compared to pre-CAH levels; 3) the same as before conversion to CAH; 4) expanded in scope compared to pre-CAH levels; and 5) added as a new service following conversion. We compared the four hospital subgroups to examine whether linkage or affiliation history had an impact on post-conversion scope of services (see Tables 3 and 4). The five hospital services that had the most post-conversion change included general inpatient surgery, obstetrical services, inpatient rehabilitation services, outpatient surgery, and outpatient specialty clinics. Each of these services was less influenced by system linkages than pre-conversion affiliation agreements. For all but inpatient rehabilitation services, provision of the service prior to conversion was more likely if there had not been a pre-conversion affiliation agreement. The relationship between pre-conversion affiliation agreements and post-conversion scope of services warrants further scrutiny in future analyses.

TABLE 3

Post-CAH Scope of Inpatient and Outpatient Services by Hospital Linkage and Pre-Conversion Network Affiliation Agreement History

	Pre-CAH (%)	*Post-CAH Change*		
		Same (%)	*New/Expand (%)*	*Limit/Drop (%)*
General Surgery				
FS* with agreement (n=72)	51	83	8	8
FS w/o agreement (n=45)	71	76	9	15
Sys/CM** with agreement (n=69)	51	78	9	13
Sys/CM w/o agreement (n=25)	76	80	8	12
Obstetrics				
FS with agreement (n=72)	22	90	4	6
FS w/o agreement (n=45)	44	82	4	13
Sys/CM with agreement (n=70)	26	90	3	7
Sys/CM w/o agreement (n=25)	60	84	0	16
Inpatient Rehab				
FS with agreement (n=72)	65	83	15	1
FS w/o agreement (n=45)	60	91	9	0
Sys/CM with agreement (n=69)	54	88	10	1
Sys/CM w/o agreement (n=25)	52	80	20	0
Outpatient Surgery				
FS with agreement (n=68)	65	76	25	4
FS w/o agreement (n=45)	89	69	22	9
Sys/CM with agreement (n=70)	66	63	26	11
Sys/CM w/o agreement (n=25)	88	64	24	12
Outpatient Specialty				
FS with agreement (n=72)	79	67	31	3
FS w/o agreement (n=45)	89	69	29	2
Sys/CM with agreement (n=70)	81	67	30	3
Sys/CM w/o agreement (n=25)	84	78	28	0

* FS = freestanding

** Sys/CM = system or contract-managed

TABLE 4

Post-CAH Scope of Support and Sub-Acute Care Service by Hospital Linkage and Pre-Conversion Network Affiliation Agreement History

	Pre-CAH (%)	*Post-CAH Change*		
		Same (%)	*New/Expand (%)*	*Limit/Drop (%)*
General Surgery				
FS* with agreement (n=72)	51	83	8	8
FS w/o agreement (n=45)	71	76	9	15
Sys/CM** with agreement (n=69)	51	78	9	13
Sys/CM w/o agreement (n=25)	76	80	8	12
Obstetrics				
FS with agreement (n=72)	22	90	4	6
FS w/o agreement (n=45)	44	82	4	13
Sys/CM with agreement (n=70)	26	90	3	7
Sys/CM w/o agreement (n=25)	60	84	0	16
Inpatient Rehab				
FS with agreement (n=72)	65	83	15	1
FS w/o agreement (n=45)	60	91	9	0
Sys/CM with agreement (n=69)	54	88	10	1
Sys/CM w/o agreement (n=25)	52	80	20	0
Outpatient Surgery				
FS with agreement (n=68)	65	76	25	4
FS w/o agreement (n=45)	89	69	22	9
Sys/CM with agreement (n=70)	66	63	26	11
Sys/CM w/o agreement (n=25)	88	64	24	12
Outpatient Specialty				
FS with agreement (n=72)	69	67	31	3
FS w/o agreement (n=45)	89	69	29	2
Sys/CM with agreement (n=70)	81	67	30	3
Sys/CM w/o agreement (n=25)	84	72	28	0

* FS = freestanding

** Sys/CM = system or contract-managed

Inpatient general surgical and obstetrical services appeared to lose the most ground after conversion, with 25 hospitals losing some form of surgical capacity (11 dropped and 14 limited) and 19 hospitals losing some obstetrical capacity (17 dropped and 2 limited). Inpatient rehabilitation services, on the other hand, demonstrated a net gain in capacity across the sample, with eight hospitals adding new services, 19 expanding existing services and only one hospital dropping and one hospital limiting services.

Service capacity was improved for outpatient surgery, where four hospitals added, 47 expanded and only six dropped services, and for specialty clinics, where five hospitals added new services, 53 expanded existing services and only four limited and one dropped services. There were significant increases in capacity for the two support services of radiology and laboratory. Radiological services were expanded in 53 hospitals and limited in only two, and laboratory services were added to one hospital, expanded in 42 and limited in only one.

Swing bed services demonstrated a slight gain, perhaps reflecting the common strategy of either adding swing bed services before seeking designation or combining a swing bed application with the application to convert to a CAH. The largest drop in availability of services involved home health services, most likely due to the implementation of a Prospective Payment System (PPS) for home health services.

Hospital Networking Experiences

A specific condition of participation in the Flex Programme is that a state must establish at least one rural health network. At a minimum, the network must contain a CAH and at least one other acute care hospital with which the CAH has established an affiliation agreement for transfer and referral arrangements. Although federal guidelines could be interpreted as requiring a minimum of one network per state, most states require it for each and every CAH certified for federal designation. All but one CAH reported having a network affiliation.

The most prevalent network relationship observed at this stage of the programme has been more of a horizontal than vertical arrangement, limited mostly to a dyad link between a CAH and its "support hospital." Although the evidence is not complete, the data suggest that most of these relationships involve only a marginal expansion of pre-existing market relationships. Network affiliations that extended beyond typical open market relationships were mostly influenced directly by the strategic mission of a CAH's support hospital, or more indirectly by the organisational culture that has evolved under pre-CAH system collaboration. In the first case, the level and degree of collaborative activity would depend mostly upon the mutual interests of the CAH and its support hospital. In the latter case, the level and degree of collaborative activity would represent the sum total of inter-organisational experiences (shared history of collaboration and cooperation) that accrued prior to participation in the Flex Programme (see page 3 for discussion).

Network affiliations tend to be circumscribed by the affiliation agreements that have been formed between network participants. An exploration of the nature of these network agreements provides us with a potential window into the organisational relationships that are emerging and influencing the behaviours of CAHs and their network partners. In an attempt to gain a better understanding of these relationships, CAH administrators were asked in the telephone survey to identify the major areas of their existing affiliation agreements and indicate if these agreements had been in place prior to their conversion to CAH.

Networking Lessons

The degree of network development witnessed during the second year of the Flex Programme has been more limited than we expected. The networks that have emerged within the programme generally have been crafted to meet the minimum requirements of the federal and state guidelines and conditions for participation. However, during our site visits to the participating states we observed several examples of network development occurring outside the minimum requirements (e.g., the peer review and credentialing networks that have developed in states such as North Dakota and Kansas).

These observations provide credence to the adage "form follows function." They do not speak specifically to the effectiveness of the Flex Programme in fostering effective rural health network development. However, they are consistent with the overwhelming influence of a long history of rural health market crises on the ability of key stakeholders to focus their efforts and decide which priorities should receive the limited resources available to rural areas.

The majority of network relationships formed through participation in the Flex Programme were with an affiliated hospital. Such connections were expressly outlined in both federal and state programme guidelines, and participants suggested that they were a significant factor in conversion success and in achieving organisational change. They provided planning expertise, financial support, staff assistance, administrative expertise, clinical expertise, and equipment to the CAHs when they most needed them.

These observations indicate the need for CAH administrators and staff to pay careful attention to the relationships they choose to develop with a support hospital. Most of the comments provided by CAH administrators referred to effectively nurturing relationships with their support hospital and not with fellow network participants.

Larger Facilities Need to See Smaller CAHs as Partners

These comments from CAH administrators point to ways in which the support facility can interact with the CAH so as to minimize fears about loss of autonomy. It can "give CAHs the sense that they are in charge and that support hospitals are facilitating their development." The more flexible the larger hospital's management team, the easier this balance is to achieve. However, it does not depend solely upon the relationships that develop between the administrators. "Relationships must begin at the physician level so that they are ready and willing to conduct outreach efforts with the smaller hospital's medical staff." The administrators must be in tune with each other, but if the physicians are not, the whole effort can be undermined.

The CAH management team often must explore ways to educate the support hospitals (especially middle management) as to what is involved in running a CAH and how operations need to be configured. A potential trouble spot is an increase in errors related to transfers between the support hospital and the CAH.

A CAH's selection of an affiliate hospital is a cornerstone of the Flex Programme. However, the development of effective network affiliations between CAHs and support hospitals has been limited. Although some CAHs receive significant benefits from their support hospital affiliations both in terms of services and access to capital resources, many CAHs do not.

There are a variety of possible explanations for why some hospitals currently are not involved in effective network affiliations. For example, hospital administrators may have had their hands full with pending financial crises and needed to focus on CAH conversion as quickly as possible for financial relief. Other hospitals, by virtue of their leadership, organisational culture, or history, may never have been interested in network membership and did not find sufficient incentive in the Flex Programme to change their attitudes.

Successful affiliations are more likely when the need is evident, intentions are known and expectations are clear. Bringing these ingredients together and convening potential partners takes time and energy. At this point in time, it is impossible to determine the potential benefit of a supportive network affiliation for the conversion and operation of CAHs. We know that some network relationships work very well but we don't know if the ingredients of their success can be generalized to other environments. We expect that as CAHs stabilize their finances it will become easier to identify how network relationships may play a supportive role. Our observations of rural health networks to date suggest that the most likely form that post-conversion affiliations will take is that of a horizontal network (i.e., hospital to hospital) and that the most likely way that non-acute care providers will be involved will be through their existing corporate ties with the hospitals involved in the network. The degree to which CAH network forms may differ will depend largely upon the existence of market incentives (e.g., revenue opportunities, regulatory relief, and state guidance).

Pick Your Partner Carefully

CAH administrators need to examine the potential relationships with their support hospitals very carefully to ensure that the growing relationship is based on clear understandings and expectations. For example, one hospital that we visited this year had an affiliate hospital that was helpful in encouraging specialists to travel to the CAH for clinics. The community benefited from the increase in access to specialty services, and the CAH received a secondary benefit from increased community satisfaction with availability of services. However, the financial benefits for the CAH were less clear. The specialists were given free use of clinic space and billed patients out of their home offices rather than through the CAH. The increase in specialty services appears to have had little impact on the CAH's inpatient volume, and some patients are choosing to drive to the more distant hospital for follow-up and additional services.

The relationship should not be solely based on fulfilling the Flex Programme guidelines. "Get specifics on what the relationship will provide"... and when you get close to setting the terms, get it in writing. A successful relationship between a CAH and its support hospital "needs to be two ways...benefiting both members of the partnership...a financial connection work(s) best." With minimal effort one can translate financial aspects into a benefit or cost. However, non-financial connections will also work if they can be translated into measurable outcomes for the partners involved.

The Decision to Network May Be Difficult

For some, the realisation that collaborating with one or more area providers could result in mutual benefits was new. There are still many small rural hospitals whose administrators, board members and/or medical staff delay collaborative ventures for fear of losing organisational or practice-related autonomy. One CAH administrator noted that "indecision is a decision." Leadership is just as important for network development as it is for managing the conversion of a CAH, and indecision is not a leadership quality. Success for the CAH administrator depends upon the ability to understand and grasp opportunities to further secure organisational linkages that are beneficial to the CAH. "You need a good strong tertiary care partner...to make it work and most of the time you have to sell the bargain to the support hospital - you can't do that from a position of fear and mistrust."

Some Environments are More Fertile than Others

A number of respondents noted that sometimes you can just be lucky to find yourself in a social environment that supports the development of collaborative relationships. For example, some locales have a natural "shared spirit and identity" that can jumpstart collaborative ventures. In other cases, the administrators or various providers may have had the opportunity to develop close personal ties with each other (this may be more common in situations where providers already share an organisational linkage through a system or management contract). Our site visits uncovered a number of examples of networks that developed because of internal, shared interests and visions of provider administrators. In one case a number of CAHs worked together on quality issues involving peer review. In another site, the close personal ties between hospital chief executive officers (CEOs) made it possible to move smoothly toward a more collaborative structure for several CAHs that might otherwise have gone their separate ways. The support hospital was afforded some protection against encroachment from other larger hospitals, while the smaller hospitals received access to a teleconferencing system, EKG reading support, billing and coding support, equipment purchases, cardiology support and specialty physician clinics. The support hospital is running a training programme that can be used by the CAHs in the network for radiology technicians and emergency room (ER) nurse training. A more tacit benefit that was unexpected was the increased presence that these hospitals gained in relation to the state hospital association. These represent opportunities for collaborative ventures and networking success to foster continuing efforts with increasing degrees of investment/commitment to the continued operation and survival of a network.

ACHIEVEMENTS AND BACKGROUND

By solid co-operation between national and provincial health departments, supported by others inside and outside government, a national health system has been created.

Achievements

The following summary reflects the key achievements since 1994:

- Outlining of the government's health policies through the tabling of the White Paper on the Transformation of the Health System in April 1997.
- The elimination of discriminatory structures and practices in the public health system.
- Consolidation of fourteen fragmented health administrations inherited from the apartheid system into a national and nine provincial health departments.
- Transformation of the public health system from a fragmented, racially divided hospital-centred service to an integrated, comprehensive national service that emphasises the health needs of disadvantaged people especially those living in rural areas.
- Expansion of the primary care infra-structure:
    - Since 1994 more than 700 new clinics have been built or had major upgrading (495 of which were completely newly built);

- 2298 existing clinics have received new equipment and were upgraded;
- 124 new visiting points were built; and
- 125 new mobile clinics purchased.

— Health care, free at the point of delivery, for pregnant and lactating women, children under the age of six years and all who use the public primary health care system was introduced.

— Introduction of the Integrated Management of Childhood Illnesses (IMCI), with training of health workers.

— The provision of primary school nutrition services through which about 5 million children have benefited and many employment opportunities have been created in communities.

— Major progress achieved with the implementation of the district health system through the demarcation of interim health districts and the setting up of the regional and district offices.

— Launching of the National Drug Policy in 1996 and the development of essential drug lists and standard treatment guidelines for primary health care and hospital levels (paediatric and adult levels of care) and some improvement in the availability of essential drugs in public facilities.

— Realignment of tenders in line with the essential drug lists.

— Introduced the World Health Organisation recommended Direct Observed Treatment Short-course (DOTS) strategy to combat TB in 1996.

— Employment of 402 Cuban and 44 other foreign doctors to strengthen hospital based care for rural communities and to provide proper support to our primary health system.

— The introduction of community service for newly graduating South African doctors.

— An impressive record in transforming health legislation. Acts have been passed to:

- Rationalise Health Professions Councils and make them more representative of the South African population;
- Make drugs more available and affordable in the country;
- Promote the use of generic products;
- More effectively regulate the medical schemes industry;
- Enable safe and legal termination of pregnancies in public and private facilities;
- Warn the public of the dangers of smoking; and
- Limit smoking in public places and ban the advertising of tobacco products.
- Commencement of a system of inquiries into maternal deaths to ensure the prevention of unnecessary deaths.
- Implementation of the Choice on Termination of Pregnancy Act, 1996, with the training of midwives in termination of pregnancy, and in post-abortion counselling.
- Training of advanced midwives and facilitators for most provinces.
- Prioritisation of the health of children has ensured that South Africa is firmly on the road to polio free certification and the achievement of a

significant decline in measles due to mass immunisation campaigns.

- Introduction of Hepatitis B vaccine in April 1995 and HiB vaccine in July 1999.
- Advanced preparations for the establishment of a Telemedicine network including 28 pilot sites in the public health system by July 1999 to enhance access to expertise and resources in rural areas.
- Carried out the first ever hospital audit in South Africa in 1996, which resulted in the introduction of the hospital rehabilitation programme.
- Carried out a cost centre study as the first step in the implementation of a system of decentralized management to promote greater efficiency in our hospitals.
- Launch of "Partnerships Against AIDS" by Deputy President Mbeki in October 1998 to intensify efforts aimed at arresting the epidemic and the development of the Government AIDS Action Plan under the auspices of the Inter Ministerial Committee on HIV/AIDS.
- Conducted the first ever "Demographic and Health Survey" in South Africa that provides a reliable baseline for monitoring health status change.

Background

Prior to 1994 the South African health system was built on apartheid ideology and characterised by racial and geographic disparities, fragmentation and duplication and hospi-centricism with lip service paid to the primary health care approach. There were 14 Departments of Health each having their own objectives. Access to health care for rural communities and those classified as 'black' was difficult. Besides the lack of facilities, the financial burden of finding and financing transport to health facilities and payment for health services acted as barriers to access to care. Many rural hospitals had very limited access to medical doctors and medicines were not always available at public health facilities and expensive.

Over the past few years, our country has been through an exciting process of transformation. During this time we have benefited from the lessons of others and believe that we have also contributed to humanity's common foundation of wisdom.

We have firmly placed before our country a perspective of health that recognises good health as both a prerequisite for social and economic development as well as an outcome of that process. Health must be considered as an investment rather than simply as expenditure. It is also a perspective that sees good health as a product of many determinants - many of which lie outside the formal health sector. For our country to succeed and our citizens to be healthy - government and all associated institutions cannot and should not function in isolation. Our inability to form strong partnerships has been one of our key weaknesses as a government over the past 5 years, a weakness that must be urgently corrected.

It is common knowledge that lack of water and sanitation is a common cause of cholera, diarrhoeal and other illnesses that afflict so many in our country and that there is a relationship between various communicable diseases, including TB, and conditions of squalor. Yet we often have not structured our institutions and service delivery systems in ways that can easily respond to these realities. The adoption by this government of the Primary Health Care Approach forces us to challenge this model. We share the vision captured in the President's "State of the Nation" address - a vision of integrated planning and delivery. This is the only way to optimise use of resources and derive the full utility of our investments.

In spite of these shortcomings, we believe we have made significant gains in the past five years. By solid co-operation between national and provincial health departments, supported by others inside and outside government, a national health system has been created. The policy of Primary Health Care was clearly enunciated and now commands national support. The public health system has been transformed from a fragmented, racially divided, hospital-centred service favouring the urban population into an integrated, comprehensive national service driven by the need to redress historical inequities and to give priority to the provision of essential health care to disadvantaged people, especially those residing in the rural areas.

The public health system can be proud of the structural transformation it has effected. Practical progress has also been made in filling in the details of this transformation. Hundreds of new clinics have been built or rehabilitated, and health care has been made free at the point of delivery for pregnant women, young children and all who use the public primary health care system. New posts have been created at the public primary level of care. The access of poor people to essential health care has thereby been greatly improved. The policy of the delivery of primary health care through the district health system has been clearly formulated and implementation has commenced.

Inevitably, a multitude of challenges remain: planning and management skills are still weak at all levels, but especially in hospitals; management systems need to be upgraded; essential management information is lacking at all levels of the health system; more primary health care nurses need to be trained; the quality of care that is provided in public health facilities must be improved; many clinics are short of equipment; drug procurement, distribution and management must be improved; and the consolidation of the district health system is bedevilled by the continuing territorial divide between provincial and local governments.

We need to focus more attention on the building of a culture of quality and efficiency throughout the health care system. We need to explore possible areas of co-operation between the private and public sectors. Despite these challenges we are certain that we are well on the road to building a health service that all South Africans can be proud of.

LOCAL NETWORKING STRATEGIES USED BY CRITICAL ACCESS HOSPITALS

As community institutions, critical access hospitals (CAHs) must be responsive to the needs of their communities and the populations located within them. In recognition of this fact, the Rural Hospital Flexibility Programme (Flex Programme) contains provisions to encourage CAHs to engage in networking activities as a way of identifying and addressing local health care infrastructure problems and needs. This chapter will focus on the local networking activities in which CAHs engage and the impact of those efforts on the hospital and the local health care infrastructure.

Local community networking initiatives are often overlooked in discussions of CAH networking efforts as the focus is generally on the linkages between CAHs and larger hospitals or health care systems. Despite this tendency to underestimate the importance of local community networking activities, they can be a critical element of a CAH's efforts to connect with its community. Effective local linkages can help to develop the trust that results in the expanded use of the CAH's services and to cultivate greater political and financial support within the community. These networks can also serve as a source of information on the scope of services needed and desired by the community and its populations. In this way, successful local networking efforts can support the development of the local health care infrastructure by mobilizing the efforts of multiple community providers, and can serve to better integrate local services by cultivating relationships between these providers.

These local community networking efforts can include, but are not limited to programme or service enhancement initiatives with public health agencies, health departments, school systems, school-based clinics, physicians, rural health clinics, community health centers, dental clinics, mental health service organisations, and/or alternative health care providers. The exact mix depends on the composition of providers and agencies present in the community, their traditional roles, and the level of rapport and trust they share.

Local networking initiatives have much in common with the broader set of community development activities. The major differences are that local networks are primarily composed of health care providers and are focused specifically on maximising the functioning of available health resources and building new services as dictated by community needs. Community development initiatives, in comparison, are likely to include a broader range of stakeholders (e.g., business and community leaders, consumers, and local government officials, as well as health care providers) and activities, including a broader array of public health functions. We would expect to see local networks engaged in identifying and developing new services that are needed, identifying and reaching out to underserved populations, and addressing access barriers such as transportation, geography, or language.

We did not expect to find a great deal of local networking activity despite the expectations of some federal and state officials that CAHs will engage in this type of activity under the Flex Programme. Our expectations were based on three factors which were confirmed by our observations during our Year 01 site visits. First, incentives for local networking have not been especially strong nor clear except in states like North Carolina or Michigan. Second, many hospital administrators and boards still define their hospitals by their inpatient activities. Finally, issues of short-term financial survival and/or the conversion process tend to occupy the attention of the administrators of struggling institutions. We did, however, find interesting examples in selected states such as Michigan, New Mexico, North Carolina, and West Virginia.

In an effort to better understand the nature of local networking efforts, the barriers to undertaking local networking initiatives at both the state and hospital levels, and the benefits both to CAHs and their communities, we have focused on this issue as a major component of our Year 02 study. We explored the following questions:

1. To what extent are CAHs engaged in local networking?
2. What local providers and agencies are participating in local networks?
3. To what extent are these local networks engaged in efforts to assess and address community needs?
4. What other activities are these local networks engaged in?

5. How are CAHs benefiting from participation in these efforts?
6. To what extent have these local networks strengthened local health care infrastructures?

In an effort to answer these questions, we drew on data collected from our telephone survey of 217 CAHs along with interviews with administrators, staff, and community representatives from 40 CAHs conducted during Years 01 and 02 and follow-up interviews with informants from the 24 CAHs visited in Year 01.

Survey of CAH Administrators

In the winter of 2000, the University of Minnesota completed telephone surveys of the administrators of 217 of the 239 hospitals that had been designated as Critical Access Hospitals as of September 1, 2000. The survey asked a series of questions about local networking including the types of networking activities taking place, the number of meetings between the CAH and local providers, and the degree to which CAHs are working with various players to determine community needs. Findings include:

- Most networking efforts are of the inter-community type, between CAHs and their affiliate hospitals.
- Relatively little formal networking is taking place between CAHs and local providers.
- When local networking does occur, it is generally focused on public health or social support activities and efforts to identify the health care needs of the community.

Administrators were asked "how often do you meet with representatives of local public health, mental health, emergency medical service (EMS), and/or other similar community-based health care providers that were not formally affiliated with the hospital prior to becoming a CAH?" About a third reported meeting monthly or more often, another third met quarterly, and the last third met rarely if at all (Table 5). Although more than two-thirds of the responding administrators reported meeting with local providers on a quarterly or more frequent basis before conversion, the design of our survey did not allow respondents to indicate either the format or content of those meetings.

TABLE 5

Frequency of Meetings with Local Community Providers Before Conversion

Frequency of Meetings	*N*	%
Never	13	7
Annually	16	8
Semi-annually	34	17
Quarterly	67	34
Monthly	62	31
2+ times per month	7	4

Source: 2000 Survey of CAH Administrators.

As a follow up to this question, the respondents were asked if there had been any change in the level of community provider contacts since conversion to a CAH. Seventy five percent reported that the level of contact with community providers remained about the same. In comparison, 21 percent reported more contact and 4 percent reported less contact since conversion.

The administrators were also asked to identify the extent to which they worked with various types of providers in any planning or assessment efforts to identify the health care needs of their local community. The result are summarized in Table 6. Forty three percent reported working with their affiliate hospitals to identify community needs.

The strategies used by CAHs and their affiliate hospitals to identify local health care needs included: 1) combined community needs assessments; 2) surveys, focus groups, and other data collection efforts; 3) strategic planning initiatives; 4) specialty care development; and 5) local and regional networking.

Nineteen percent worked with other health care providers with whom the CAH has long-term agreements or affiliations to identify community health care needs. The strategies employed under these networking arrangements included: 1) performing community needs assessments; 2) engaging in joint ventures/service development; 3) networking arrangements for sharing and analysing data; 4) participating in consortiums or task forces; and 5) linking with local agencies and health departments.

Finally, 39 percent reported working with local providers with which the CAH did not have long-term agreements or affiliations to identify community needs. The strategies included: 1) participating in consortiums or task forces composed of community agencies; 2) conducting community needs assessments; 3) collecting, sharing, and analysing data; and 4) the internal identification needs and/or problems. The responses to these questions are not mutually exclusive and some CAHs work with more than one category of providers to identify local health care needs.

TABLE 6

CAH Network Partners in Identifying Local Health Care Needs

Network Partners	*N*	%
Affiliate Hospital	92	43
Other Affiliated Providers	41	19
Local Non-Affiliated Providers	84	39

Source: 2000 Survey of CAH Administrators.

In an effort to determine the frequency of local community networking activities and the extent of the activities that occur under these networking arrangements, administrators were asked about a wide range of potential collaborative activities as well as the type of entities with which they collaborated around each activity. Table 7 summarizes their responses about the extent to which hospitals participated in these types of collaborative activities prior to conversion to a CAH.

TABLE 7

Collaborative Activities by Type of Collaborative Partner

Service N	*N*	*Affiliate Hospital %*	*Other Affiliated Provider (%)*	*Local Non-Affiliated Provider (%)*	*Distant Non-Affiliated Provider (%)*	*Percentage of Total Respon dents (%)*
Contract Management	72	68	24	4	4	33
Financial Services	86	76	22	0	2	40
Administrative Support	118	64	26	2	9	54
Marketing/Community Relations	54	70	22	2	6	25
MIS/Clinical Info. Systems	73	74	21	0	6	34
Primary Care Medical	54	78	17	0	6	25
Specialty Medical	148	65	7	4	24	68
Clinical Support	84	71	10	6	13	39
Quality Management	108	85	11	1	3	50
Social Support	44	55	16	23	7	20
Public Health	57	23	5	68	4	26

Source: 2000 Survey of CAH Administrators.

As can be seen from this table, the majority of collaborative efforts undertaken by CAHs involved their affiliate hospital and other providers with whom the CAH had formal affiliation agreements prior to conversion. The two service lines in which a significant amount of local networking took place prior to conversion were public health and social support activities. Of the 57 CAHs whose administrators indicated that they are collaborating around public health services, 68 percent were working with local, non-affiliated providers. Of the CAHs that engage in collaborative social support activities such as long-term care, case management, and mental health, 23 percent reported that they were networking with local non-affiliated providers.

Administrators were also asked if any affiliated or non-affiliated health care providers had made a significant contribution to identified changes in scope of services since conversion to a CAH. Only 5 CAHs out of 217 (slightly more than 2%) indicated that either kind of partner had made a significant contribution to the CAH's changes in scope of services. The providers identified included two hospitals, two specialty clinics, and a programme offering obstetric (OB) nurse training. Of these five CAHs, only two indicated that a non-affiliated local provider had contributed to the hospital's scope of services changes. In contrast, 24 percent reported that their affiliate hospital played a major role in accomplishing their reported scope of service changes.

TABLE 8

Organisations Playing a Key Role in QA/QI Capacity Since Conversion to a CAH*

	N	%
Affiliate Hospital	126	58
Other Local Providers	23	11
Public Agencies (DOH, DSS)	28	13
Clinics/Health Center	15	7
Tertiary Medical Center	22	10
Other	22	10

Source: 2000 Survey of CAH Administrators.

* These figures exceed 100 percent as the survey allowed for multiple responses to this question.

Finally, administrators were asked to identify the networking roles related to quality assurance and quality improvement initiatives. Table 8 summarizes their responses.

Not surprisingly, 58 percent of the respondents identified their affiliate hospitals as playing a key role in the improvement or refinement of their quality assurance (QA) and/or quality improvement (QI) capacity since conversion to a CAH. Ten percent named tertiary medical centers as important participants in the process. A similar number worked with a wide variety of organisations such as network and system partners, state hospital associations, management companies, EMS units, and other clinical providers around quality initiatives. Local community organisations including local providers (11%), public agencies such as the Departments of Health or Social Services (13%), and clinics/health centers (7%) were identified as participants in QA/QI activities. Of those CAHs that indicated that more than one organisation played a key role, 69 percent named their affiliate hospitals as playing the most important networking role in improvements to their QA/QI initiatives (Table 9). Other local providers and clinics/health centers were mentioned as the most important network partners by only three percent and two percent of the respondents respectively.

TABLE 9

Most Important Networking Partners in QA/QI Improvements

	N	%
Affiliate Hospital	73	69
Other Local Providers	3	3
Public Agencies (DOH, DSS)	14	13
Clinics/Health Center	2	2
Tertiary Medical Center	5	5
Other	9	9

Source: 2000 Survey of CAH Administrators.

Members of the Tracking Team have visited twenty states and forty critical access hospitals in the first two years of the Tracking Project. During the second year of the Tracking Project, the team incorporated questions on local networking initiatives into the site visit protocols in order to expand on the data obtained through the telephone survey of CAH administrators and to understand how these efforts may be implemented at the hospital level. Similar questions were posed to the administrators of the CAHs visited in Year 01 during follow-up interviews conducted during the spring of 2001. Findings from the site visits include:

- Despite interesting examples of local networking in some states, CAHs generally have not been actively involved with local community agencies/providers in efforts to address community health needs and problems.
- The local networking efforts described by administrators focus on process indicators (e.g., meetings with local providers and collaboration on needs assessments) rather than outcomes and results (e.g., the development of new services, increase in patients referrals, etc.).
- Local networking efforts typically include local health departments and/or community service agencies.

While we did not see a consistent pattern of local networking activity across the states we visited, there are states and CAHs that have undertaken promising initiatives with the potential to stimulate community-level health system change and development. These initiatives provide examples of the value of local networking and can serve to stimulate the thinking of other CAHs in the development of their own local networking plans, and that of state policy makers as they seek to encourage CAHs to become more involved in their communities.

State-Level Initiatives

A number of states, including Idaho, Kansas, Michigan, North Carolina, North Dakota, Oregon, Tennessee, and West Virginia, strongly encourage CAHs to work with local agencies and providers to address community health needs under the Flex Programme. Most typically, CAHs are expected to conduct community needs assessments in conjunction with local agencies and providers or participate as members of local coalitions of providers and agencies.

Oregon and Tennessee strongly emphasized their support for local networking initiatives in their interviews with the Tracking Team. Despite this fact, there was little local networking activity in the CAH communities that we visited. Oregon has created a programme known as CHIP which stands for Community Health Improvement Partnerships. The goal of CHIP is to create local community health networks of up to thirty members representing both direct health resources as well as community, social, and economic agencies. Oregon has hired a nationally recognized expert in the field of rural community development to assist communities in developing their health care delivery systems. Flex Programme grant dollars have been committed to the development of these networks in CAH and potential CAH communities. Despite the availability of grant dollars to support these initiatives, CHIP was not active in either of the two communities/CAHs visited.

Tennessee supports a series of regional Community Health Councils (CHCs) which are formal (state-staffed) organisations that engage in an intense community needs assessment process called Community Diagnosis. CHCs evolved from relatively informal grass-roots organisations. All 95 Tennessee counties have engaged in the Community Diagnosis process. The Tennessee Hospital Association, which administers the Flex Programme, coordinates with CHC to provide the most current and relevant health data possible to inform the CAH decision making process. Both hospitals we visited described close relationships with the CHCs in their regions. However, little actual local networking appeared to be taking place.

Kansas's Office of Local and Rural Health is attempting to shift the focus of its rural health networks to more population-based activities. In this way, it hopes to target populations that fall through the cracks of the service system and provide a structure for local providers to work together. Kansas has been struggling with this issue as the majority of CAH/network projects have not been using the community-focused strategies described in the state health plan. Representatives from the state office of rural health described the difficulty of shifting the traditional horizontal hospital networks to community-based networks. They explained that horizontal networks are not structured to make these types of transitions naturally. It is their hope that they will be able to facilitate the transition by separating community development activities from network development activities in a way that makes it more attractive for all interested parties, and allows the participants to focus on specific outcomes of networking rather than the relationships themselves.

Idaho has been working with three communities to pilot a network enhancement project. The communities of St. Marie's, American Falls, and Weiser are initiating network development beyond the common hospital-to-hospital model and will include community health centers, public health districts, rural health clinics, and possibly the local justice and/or education systems. It will be a test to see if the state can effectively enhance system integration at the local level through the use of grants to encourage broader participation.

Staff from the New Mexico Office of Rural Health stated that local community networking is an important priority and that there is an urgent need to integrate private clinics, public health, EMS, community health centers, and mental health providers. Nonetheless, agencies in one community we visited have been engaged in strong, long-standing rivalries with each other. State offices that commit to helping communities resolve these conflicts face a daunting task, and need resources and time to have an impact. Few state offices are, at this point, equipped to work on these issues.

Michigan encourages local networking by funding the development of Multi-Purpose Collaborative Bodies (MPCBs) throughout the state. CAHs are encouraged to actively participate in these groups. MPCBs are community-based groups composed of a broad array of service providers and agencies that meet regularly to discuss local coordination and service issues. The state has also broadened its definition of networking in the second year of the Flex Programme to include a variety of community-based health care providers and health care related organisations. One official from the Michigan Center for Rural Health conceptualizes these networks as a series of concentric circles with the hospital in the center, physicians and nurses in the next ring, and agencies such as public health and the United Way in the outer ring. Despite the state's emphasis on this concept, they admitted that it is catching on more slowly than expected and that most CAH networking efforts have occurred between hospitals.

The North Carolina Office of Rural Health also emphasizes linkages between local providers and CAHs. As part of the conversion process, CAHs must commit to working with local providers (including public health), supporting the continuation of necessary community services, and providing services to vulnerable populations. Staff from the state office of rural health estimate that 60 to 70 percent of the agendas for local networking efforts developed by CAHs are determined by the needs of the communities in which they are located. The remainder of their agendas are determined by the institutional interests of the CAHs themselves.

West Virginia's criteria for the distribution of Flex Programme grants emphasize community needs assessments and community involvement although the staff explained that these initiatives play out differently from hospital to hospital. West Virginia has placed major emphasis on network building in its mini-grant programme. Despite this state-level emphasis, concerns have been raised about the networks developed under a rural managed care center grant during the period 1994 through 1999 as they have not proven to be self-sustaining. One source suggested that network building for its own sake is a poor investment.

CAH/Community-Level Initiatives

One hospital that we visited in New Mexico described a local perinatal providers' group that meets monthly and includes nurses from the OB unit, midwives, physicians, a nurse practitioner from an Indian Health Service clinic, and a nurse practitioner who staffs a local clinic. In addition, a local maternal and child health coalition for perinatal enrichment meets monthly with representatives from Women, Infants, and Children (WIC), Medicaid, Families First (a programme of the public health department), and the mental health department. These meetings serve to provide a sort of case management role for an at-risk population.

In northern Michigan, one CAH has entered into a formal agreement with the county health department to provide culposcopy and mammography services to health department clients. They also sponsored a women's health day, also in conjunction with the county health department, that attracted 35 women from the community. The same hospital has also worked with local tribes to develop additional women's services in the community. The hospital provided the necessary physician and clinical staff and the tribes purchased equipment necessary to develop those services. The hospital's administrator and other key staff participate in the local human services collaborative board (the area's MPCB). The board meets monthly to discuss local coordination and service issues and includes representatives from the hospital, local health care and social service agencies, the health department, and the community mental health center. These activities resulted in increased utilisation of the hospital's outpatient services and the development of new services for residents of the community. These outreach efforts also generated increased political support for the hospital. This support was particularly important when the renewal of its county tax support came up for vote. According to the administrator, a positive decision by the voters was far from guaranteed.

A CAH in central North Carolina is exploring public health collaborations as its emphasis shifts from increasing market share to improving access for county residents. The hospital's relationship with the health department began with the joint development of minority crisis intervention services as well as programmes and services targeting the growing population of Hmong and Laotian refugees settling in its area. Another CAH in North Carolina has entered into a close relationship with the local health department in which it meets regularly with and supports part of the salary of the Director. This relationship was undertaken at the direction of the North Carolina Office of Rural Health and has resulted in a closer linkage of the hospital to the needs of the community. It has also allowed the hospital to support the local public health system in the face of recent budget cuts in North Carolina. The same hospital is also developing a diabetes programme that pulls in other providers, a nurse triage programme that provides off hour coverage for local physicians (thereby strengthening the relationship between the physicians and the hospital), and a school nurse programme with the local schools which the school department has committed to supporting after the initial demonstration grant expires. This hospital's local networking efforts have resulted in increased inpatient and outpatient utilisation as well as the maintenance of key public health functions within the county.

A West Virginia CAH has worked with a local school to develop a successful school-based clinic that is open to students and staff of the school system and their families. The clinic has been well received and treats all patients regardless of ability to pay. The hospital is currently planning to develop a clinic with a school system in an adjoining community to expand the availability of primary care services in surrounding areas. This same hospital is involved with a regional network that includes hospitals, clinics, community health centers, and birthing centers. The expanded membership has created some difficulties for the network as it is difficult to meet the diverse needs of the participants. Some fallout in membership has occurred as the hospital members perceive their needs are not being met. The hospital has also attempted to work more closely with the local Federally-Qualified Health Center (FQHC). The hospital would like to serve as the FQHC's lab vendor believing that it can offer quicker turnaround and lower costs. To date, the FQHC has rejected the hospital's proposal due to its (the FQHC's) desire to remain autonomous. Despite this fact, the relationship between the institutions seems solid as the family physicians at the FQHC perform most of the deliveries in the hospital's OB unit. The hospital and the FQHC worked together to conduct surveys and analyse data as part of a needs assessment undertaken by the hospital during its conversion. This hospital reports greater outpatient utilisation within the community as well as the ability to raise significant dollars from the community ($310,000) to equip its new addition which houses it emergency room and Rural Health Clinic. It has also resulted in an expansion of services to students and staff (as well as their families) of the school in which the school-based clinic is located. Community officials have also linked the hospital to their ability to recruit and retain industry.

Before leaving this section, it will be useful to discuss (and refute) some common responses to our site visit questions about local networking efforts. Administrators often described situations in which members of their physician, nursing, or physical therapy staff were employed by local agencies (health departments, family planning programmes, etc.) or providers (nursing homes, home health agencies, etc.). Conversely, they also described situations in which staff from these agencies and/or providers worked at the hospital. In exploring these relationships, it became clear that these were independent and private arrangements rather than strategic organisational collaborations. Although these linkages serve to develop some individual familiarity with local services on the part of the participating health professionals, rarely have they resulted in any changes to the local infrastructure.

Another common description of local networking provided by administrators was the systematic referral of patients to local home health agencies, nursing homes, mental health agencies, federally qualified health agencies, rural health clinics, etc. Referral of patients does not constitute a formal effort to develop new services, address access issues, or reach out to an underserved population.

A third common response was that, while no formal linkages and networking efforts were taking place at the local level between the hospital and other agencies/providers, the size and closeness of the community meant that key staff from the hospital and these organisations all knew each other and had frequent contact at various social and community functions. By virtue of these informal contacts, it was suggested that the key stakeholders in the community were aware of local access and service needs. Rarely do these "social" contacts have the impact typically ascribed to them, however, as they tend to be sporadic, unstructured, and occur in the context of some other event.

Finally, administrators tended to discuss local networking in terms of the variety of activities participated in (e.g., the number of meetings with community providers attended, the task forces served on, the needs assessments and analysis of local data conducted as part of the conversion application, etc.), rather than the attainment of specific objectives or goals. Too often, these activities, particularly meetings and task forces, seemed to be oriented more towards keeping track of the players than the accomplishment of specific tasks and goals.

Discussions and Recommendations

These characterisations of local networking efforts serve to underscore common misconceptions about networking efforts in general and local networking efforts in particular. Discussions of networking initiatives too often focus on the process of networking rather than outcomes. In other words, the focus of attention is often on such things as meetings between network participants, the collection and analysis of data, and the formation of tasks forces rather than on the development of new and needed services, the expansion of access for underserved and vulnerable populations, retention and growth of local market share, and/or the reversal of patient outmigration.

It might be argued that these process-oriented activities can be thought of as preliminary steps that can facilitate the development of relationships and trust between the CAH and community providers and agencies. While this may be true to a certain extent, these process activities are not likely to foster the development of real trust unless they are focused on the attainment of specific goals and require the formal commitment of the participants. As one respondent stated, "networks work best when focused on specific task and projects."

Given the relatively limited evidence of local networking occurring between CAHs and the agencies/providers in their communities, should incentives to encourage local networking initiatives be part of state Flex Programmes? Given the potential benefits, why has there not been more activity (or more success from state initiatives)? How can states and state Flex Programmes encourage CAHs to undertake these activities? What are the potential benefits to the CAH and to the local health care infrastructure?

We would argue that the Flex Programme should have incentives to promote local networking. As discussed earlier, rural health care systems can be thought of as a series of concentric circles with the hospital at the center, if only because the hospital has the most resources and the most visible presence. Rural hospitals are generally the largest health care provider in their communities and, often, their counties. As such, they are frequently, but not always, looked to by other providers/ agencies as well as the general public for leadership and, in fact, are positioned to provide that leadership. As we have seen, CAHs too often look outside of their communities to larger hospitals and hospital systems for leadership and assistance. Although this may be appropriate around many administrative and operation functions, this external focus does little to bolster the CAH's standing as a community leader surrounding local health care issues. CAHs can and should provide leadership around the identification of community health care needs.

As to why we have not seen more local networking, a number of factors may help to explain the relatively low activity levels. Despite a ten-year effort by the American Hospital Association to move hospitals to a more community-oriented perspective, many hospital administrators still define their facilities by their inpatient activities. Moreover, the incentives provided under the Flex Programme to undertake more extensive local networking are generally quite limited. As mentioned earlier, local networking efforts are likely to take a back seat to efforts to stabilize cash flow and prepare for conversion given the relatively precarious financial positions of many CAHs. As one CAH administrator from Oklahoma explained to us, "You don't bring the guests into the kitchen before the meal is ready." Local networking has to occur in the context of the hospital's full range of obligations and activities. It may be that CAHs must stabilize their cash flow and operations before they can focus on external networking activities in which the hospital shares the responsibility for moving the process forward. Finally, local turf and political struggles may impede local networking efforts. The administrator may have to overcome bad blood that has arisen between past administrators and other agency heads. The hard feelings often long outlast the memory of the particular issue. Other local providers may resent the dominance of the CAH in their communities or fear the loss of their own autonomy as a result of engaging in local networking activities. Effective hospital leadership often involves learning how to work effectively with smaller community agencies. The CAH administrator may have to walk a very careful line to keep the process moving without appearing to dominate it. Any one (or combination) of these factors is more than sufficient to restrain local community networking efforts.

We have also seen significant benefits to the hospitals that are engaged in local networking activities that can be attributed, at least in part, to these efforts. In addition to the expanded utilisation of outpatient/ambulatory volumes, the benefits described by the hospitals include increased community and political support as well as enhanced public and private fund raising capacity. The communities in which these facilities are located have benefited by an expansion of services to their residents, a maintenance of key services, and an improved ability to recruit new industry. In at least one community, local networking efforts have resulted in the maintenance of important public health functions in the face of state budget cuts. As can be seen, these activities have resulted in a "win-win" situation for both the hospitals and their communities. Making the positive benefits apparent to all potential partners should help to advance local networking efforts.

During our site visits at the state and hospital level, we have seen that disbursement of small grants by state Flex Programmes can have a definite impact on the development of networking relationships and services. As such, state Flex Programmes should develop incentives to encourage local networking initiatives surrounding the identification of community needs and the development of specific projects and services, preferably those that address the needs of vulnerable populations or gaps in the local health care infrastructure as identified by locally driven needs assessments. The distribution of grant funds should target the accomplishment of specific and measurable goals. At the same time, the agencies responsible for administering the Flex Programme should develop the internal capacity to assist CAHs and local provider groups to work together.

In addition to the above mentioned grant funding, we would also suggest clarifying Flex Grant funding priorities at both the federal and state levels in order to explicitly promote local networking initiatives. This could be done by targeting specific health system improvements, such as the creation of new services or the development of community-level health plans, that require collaboration and community input. The development of technical assistance programmes, largely based on existing community development models, would be of help to states, communities, and hospitals as they undertake their own local networking projects. In particular, these programmes should include training in different community and network development models, group process, conflict resolution, team building, consensus building, strategic planning, and health and programme planning. This would be very useful for state officials called upon to mediate turf/boundary battles and other community level conflicts.

By taking a leadership role in the development of local networks and services, CAHs can position themselves as essential community providers. This should strengthen their relationships with their communities and local providers. Potential benefits of these strengthened relationships may include greater political and financial support (in terms of either ability to mobilize support for tax support or direct fundraising), increased patient referrals, and reductions in patient out-migration.

Take-Away Points

Despite interesting examples of local networking in selected states, many CAHs have not been actively involved with local community agencies in efforts to address community health needs and problems. Most CAHs have been inwardly preoccupied with the conversion process and short-term financial survival.

Where CAHs have engaged in local networking activities, they have tended to do so with targeted encouragement and support from state offices of rural health and hospital associations. Incentives are very important in encouraging hospitals to shift some of their focus to their local community.

Local networking efforts often fail due to process-oriented difficulties. Attention to results and outcomes is critical.

Community networking can reduce patient outmigration, increase appropriate local utilisation, help maintain key services, promote community ownership and support of the hospital, and build political support.

3

Case Study: Aspects of Hospital Enterprise Management in U.K.

CASE STUDY 1: MANAGEMENT OF CHANGE; NEW TECHNOLOGY AND ORGANISATIONAL DEVELOPMENT IN U.K. HOSPITALS

Current developments within the health services bear eloquent testimony to the fact of organisational change. This process has continued since the birth of the NHS in 1948. In itself this was a monumental change bringing all the major health agencies, except local authorities, under the umbrella of a single organisation. The result, as we have seen, was not the creation of a static body—a final solution to the Nation's health needs—but a dynamic organisation capable of undergoing change and development in response to a wide variety of factors. Some of those factors have arisen within the organisation itself as a reflection of the general social developments within society—a notably increased membership of trade unions within the NHS, for example. Others have impinged and imposed themselves from the environment: the RAWP formulae, the planning emphasis on community medicine and the introduction of high technology into health care practices. These are some of the examples that have made organisational change inevitable.

Not all change has been perceived as unequivocally

good. However, where there is a net gain, the organisation must learn to absorb the costs. For some workers change can be a painful process and involve job loss and redundancy. In other cases, life-time perceptions of working norms and practices may appear to be discounted, leaving workers emotionally stranded as their careers, together with their knowledge and skills, appear to founder on the rising tide of uncertainty.

There are some occupations for which the NHS has tended to become a collusive monopsony since, apart from London weighting, all health authorities at present are obliged to offer Whitley Council salaries and conditions to almost all staff and to refrain from the exploitation of local labour markets. (This position has been slightly relaxed to permit the appointment of the relatively small number of NHS general managers on fixed term contracts at higher rates, particularly those recruited from outside the service.) Under these circumstances, *de facto* changes in job content and status, skills and knowledge, as a result of policy decisions and/or operational requirements, are required to be accomodated by the adaptation, attitude change and retraining of staff in order to maintain employment. At the time of writing it is unclear how far-reaching in this respect will be the effects of the introduction of performance-related pay and to what extent this concept will permeate sub-general management strata. A further factor remains the uncertainty regarding the development of the 'privatization' strategy and the kind of health service that will emerge because of it.

For some this aspect of change provides an undoubted stimulus and challenge, particularly if changes are perceived as incremental and an expected and natural component of professional and career development. If training is also available, this is likely to facilitate change, but the degree of resistance may well depend upon the worker's perception of his new role and its status, given that salary is unaffected. More rapid change, as might occur with the privatization of a part of the service or the rapid introduction of new technology may give less time for personal adjustment and increase feelings of alienation at work. Although Blauner's work on alienation specifically refers to factory employees, we believe his concepts are transferable to other large organisations. We therefore use this term in his work-related sense and not in the more general sense employed by Marx.

Organisations may be either reactive or proactive—that is, planning to activate desired change rather than merely reacting to environmental impositions or client demands. The NHS has received much criticism for its reactive approach in responding to demand rather than to evaluated need and more recently this reactivity has been identified with the lack of a general management process.

As we have seen, corporate planning in health care involves the identification of need, planning how to meet that need and mobilizing the entire organisation to carry out those plans in a concerted and organised way. This cannot be achieved in a static and insensitive organisation whose members place a premium on stability or a high value on 'nostalgia' (clinging to old ways) at the expense of improved patient welfare.

The Impact of Technology

The development of technology and its applications in health care has brought enormous benefits to both patients and the organisation which serves them. Among many examples are the developments of the medical application of ultrasonics, the pacemaker, the heart-lung machine, nuclear medicine, radiology, radiotherapy, computerized scanners and laboratory analysers. The development of fibre optics has allowed a new approach to the investigation and treatment of many quite different clinical conditions with fewer 'postoperative' consequences and at a lower marginal cost than the corresponding surgery.

Some of these are clinical, high profile examples of high technology applications and health workers can no doubt identify many more less dramatic but no less significant contributions to the business of diagnosis and treatment. In terms of output, modern technology allows us to investigate and treat substantially larger numbers of patients today than, say, 30 years ago.

However, in some quarters the arrival of high technology is not always well received. In fact, it may be feared by some workers whose working practices, skills and, indeed, very employment may be threatened by its introduction. It is clear that technology itself is not to blame for this but rather the way that it is employed within the organisation. It is no solution to argue that providing redundancies are avoided there is little ground for objections to new technology. This would be to deny the intrinsic value and function of work and the social significance it gives to both individuals and groups—a point overlooked by F.W. Taylor, the father of Scientific Management.This, in essence, forms the basis of the critique of Taylor's theories by Trist who, with various co-workers from the Tavistock Institute, introduced the concept of Sociotechnical Systems. These two systems are discussed below as we identify three aspects of new technology and organisational change that are of immediate concern, namely the social consequences at work of change, deskilling and redundancy. We start by considering the influence of Taylor, recognizing that his theories are widely diffused and now form part of the culture of managerialism—the manager's right to manage—which by its unqualified stance alone has done, and continues to do, much to inhibit goodwill and mutual respect between all sections of industry.

Scientific Management

Briefly, Taylor observed that manual workers were 'inefficient', that is, they worked below maximum output because their managers either managed by guesswork or assumed that the workers knew best how tocarry out manual procedures and so left matters to them. Taylor set to work to analyse and measure in detail every movement that formed a part of each manual operation. For example, Rose reports that:

'In his studies at the Bethlehem Steel Company, Taylor discovered an optimum load in shovelling. Since the materials to be shovelled varied in their density, an entirely new range of shovels and forks had to be designed to ensure that this weight of material was always lifted. In such labouring tasks physiological fatigue could be warded off by tactically timed rest-pauses, their timing and duration depending upon the work. Study could thus determine the maximum amount of work possible in one day short of physical collapse.'

According to Taylor, defining a 'fair day's work' was a purely technical matter, being prescribed by production engineers after work-study and was therefore not a matter of opinion but science. We shall return to Taylor in our consideration of work and method study in the next chapter. Meanwhile it is sufficient to say that Taylor applied his 'scientific' principles to every aspect of work and established a major, influential and continuing 'school' of management theory. Taylor's motives were profit-oriented and he sought to reward his workers who wholly complied with his instructions with handsome bonuses directly linked to productivity. In this, however, he was largely frustrated as the company owners could not accept that any manual worker could be given the opportunity for unlimited earnings even though linked to individual productivity. In later years Taylor was to express regret since, in his attempt to alter the layout of the plant and to change the traditional way of things he was not very popular. He wrote of himself and of his work: 'I was a young man in years but I give you my word I was a great deal older than I am now, what with the worry, meanness and contemptibleness of the whole damn thing. It's a horrid life for any man to live not being able to look any workman in the face without seeing hostility there, and a feeling that every man around you is your virtual enemy.'

The Socotechnical Systems Concept

Taylor published accounts of his work in the early 1900s at about the same time as mechanization was being introduced in the British coal industry. This also involved heavily prescribing individual working methods and practices in order to accommodate the new machinery which promised to increase the productivity of every seam in which it was used. Small working groups, often family based, were required to split up and join large shifts of men. Job functions were divided between shifts so that each man and each shift was responsible for only one function and therefore the whole process was dependent upon each shift completing its allotted function on time. Productivity fell. Trist and Bamforth (an ex-miner)identified that in the introduction of new technology important social considerations had been totally ignored. They realized that coal mining with its inherent danger and discomfort was essentially a group activity with a high degree of interdependence both within and between groups. Group maintenance, therefore, is an important factor in not only productivity but in the associated problems of absenteeism, sickness, accident rates, disagreements and stoppages. When, in 1951, a mine manager in the East Midlands Division, V.W. Sheppard, initiated a composite arrangement for each shift which restored group autonomy, productivity and job satisfaction rose: absenteeism and labour turnover fell and health records improved. The essence of this experiment may be viewed as a joint optimization of both the requirements of the technology and those of the workgroup in which the group had a certain degree of autonomy.

The results of similar factory-based experiments in India and Scandinavia support this statement. In keeping with Taylor, however, the pecuniary reward system appears to be a significant ingredient as, in all these experiments, participating workers were able to earn an increase in pay. If there were lessons to be learned from the Sociotechnical Systems concept, perhaps to be transferred to areas of emerging technical innovation, they were widely ignored. In 1973, Enid Mumford could assert that:

> 'Work systems are usually designed in technical terms to meet technical and business objectives, with little thought given to the needs of people operating the system.'

It might be argued that, because this work was related to the introduction of technology into the manual production industries, the experimental evidence is irrelevant in science-based activities, including some aspects of health care. Trist disagrees. He believes that the requirement for manual dexterity is decreasing in these activities, changing the role of the worker from a doer of the work to a user and manager of the technical tools he has acquired. This is a general trend and will apply equally wherever technology displaces manual work of any kind. Hence the prescribed element of work is reduced since it is contained within the machine, whereas the discretionary part isincreased, the worker monitoring performance and intervening where necessary.Trist has stated that the reason for the workers presence:

> '... is to assess the performance of the programme and, if necessary, to change it either himself or in conjunction with others at higher levels. No longer is there 'a split at the bottom of the executive chain' which separates managers and managed. Everyone is now on the same side of the 'great divide' and whatever fences there may still be on the common side would seem best kept low. A general change is in consequence taking place in all role-relations in the enterprise. This is the underlying reason for the bureaucratic model being experienced as obsolete and maladap-tive, and also for a possible new role beginning to emerge for trade unions.'

With these brave words Trist describes here something akin to the Task Ideology of Harrison and an Ideal Type; hardly the coalition of interests that characterize the Sociotechnical Systems Concept. We would argue that where Task Ideology is dominant in an organisation we may expect to see the introduction of new technology without loss of status for the 'displaced' workers, since their role self-perception will be enhanced as will bc the degree of discretion over their working tasks. However, when 'role' or 'power' ideologies are dominant, or are significant influences in an organisation, the reverse can easily occur. In these circumstances, individual worker discretion is prescribed and handed down from above. If the skill of the worker is rendered obsolete by new technology his/her discretion, because of the organisational role definitions being related to particular skill, is perceived to have also decayed. The worker, therefore, comes to be seen as a 'button pusher' with neither skill nor discretion and with a consequent lowering of status and job satisfaction. There is also the tendency for management to impose change without consultation with the workforce or planning the change with them. This is vital if change is to be managed effectively.

We would regard the 'natural' organisational ideology or 'culture' of health teams, in operating theatres, in the community, in paramedical departments and laboratories and indeed in almost every care grouping, to be that of the Task Culture. That being so, we would expect health workers who possess both skill and knowledge to be able to evaluate new technology without fear, to adapt to its use, where appropriate, without being threatened and to enhance their role by its adoption. This means, of course that the health organisation for its part must freely acknowledge the role and worth of its workers by confirming the increased discretion that will be their natural expectation. However, the NHS has a well-developed, overall role culture prescribing job titles and role definitions and ascribing expectations of normative behaviour to employees in most occupational groups. Harrison states, 'Predictability of behaviour is high in the role-oriented organisation, and stability and respectability are often valued as much as competence. The correct response tends to be more highly valued than the effective one. Procedures for change tend to be cumbersome; therefore, the system is slow to adapt to change!'

With such institutionalized rigidity an organisation is unlikely easily to grant its imprimatur to *de facto* role development brought about by technology and in this sense one may continue to encounter, if in a milder and symbolic form, the undesirable elements that were identified by Trist and Bamforth in the longwall method of coal-getting.

There is also a strong power culture within health care which is the traditional prerogative of the medical profession. The different attitudes of the power and role orientations towards authority', says Harrison, 'might be likened to the differences between a dictatorship and a constitutional monarchy.' This is not to say that such an orientation cannot occasionally be useful both in the practice of medicine and in assisting organisational change but in general it rankles and annoys other health workers who regard themselves as co-workers with their medical colleagues but who fail to find honest reciprocation of their attitudes and views. In this 'culture' there are, by definition, winners and losers: the status of the former is gained at the expense of the latter. This is not necessarily so in other organisational ideological types. Recognition of co-workers, therefore, may become an instrument of control, is often patronizing and is scarcely going to improve relationships, and may even destroy them, as role changes because of new technology.

It is frequently identification with task ideology, as well as dedication to patient care, that provides the major maintenance factor in the service and paramedical professions of health care. Genuine and acceptable recognition is given and received within the task group from which the power ideologists tend inevitably to be excluded. Recently we have seen attempts at cultural change within the NHS through the introduction of general management and we discuss this in our final chapter. What we have endeavoured to show here is the interdependence of both the social and technical sub-systems within organisations.

De-Skilling

The second important aspect of the introduction of new technology is that of de-skilling, or the fear of it, that has long brought conflict to industrial situations. Harry Braverman advanced the thesis that de-skilling has been a dominating process in the creation of modern work organisations. Braverman was originally trained as a craftsman, a coppersmith, before becoming an editor and manager of two book publishing houses. During his 18 years as a coppersmith he saw the craftsmen being robbed of their skilled heritage as more mechanized means of production requiring less skilled, often cheaper, labour was introduced. During his time in publishing he observed the impact of computers on office skills from the 1950s onwards.

Braverman sees the detailed division of labour as the means of control, destroying whole occupations and rendering the worker inadequate for carrying through any complete production process, as occurs for example on production lines. He also sees F.W. Taylor's Scientific Management movement as a product of the need to control the activities of workers in ever-larger, monopolistic organisations. Taylor's ideas contained three main principles which are fundamental to all advanced work design, organisation and method study and industrial engineering today. These are:

- the gathering and development of knowledge of the labour processes;
- the concentration of this knowledge as an exclusive province of management;
- the use of this monopoly of knowledge to control each step of the labour process and its mode of execution.

Scientific Management concepts have thus led to the divorce of production, the manual execution of the task, from the conceptual, brain-work functions—a separation of the two essential aspects of labour. Braverman shows that people are trapped into new production methods as competitors see the need to develop similar processes to compete effectively. For example, when assembly lines were introduced at Ford's in 1913, staff turnover was some 38% for that year as workers sought employment with 'old-fashioned' car manufacturers until these also changed, or went bankrupt. Today a similar revolution has occurred in the car manufacturing industry with microprocessor driven robotic construction in Japan, Italy, USA and Britain.

Studies at Harvard have produced evidence that automation had reduced skill requirements not only of the operating workforce but occasionally of the entire factory force, including the maintenance organisation. Neither is this effect confined to craftsmen. Within the organisation Leavitt and Whisler see the impact of computers, programming and operational research on middle management roles as making them more highly structured and covered by sets of rules governing day-today decision-making. New techniques allow top management to control their middle management while top managers become more innovative and creative, particularly with programmers and R and D people moving into top positions. Because of highly programmed systems, middle managers will require, and have, less autonomy and skill.

The prediction of this statement has been moderated to some extent by economic and other factors including organisational culture and tradition. However, organisations are now poised on the threshold of an information technology explosion, which, we believe, will effect a substantial change in the way large organisations are managed. Although the capability of fulfilling Leavitt and Whisler's prophecy is at hand, new technology is likely to place more information in the hands of middle and first line managers. In the NHS, with accountability pushed downwards, if this actually occurs, the authority to act, to take decisions and to manage must be similarly delegated. Junior managers are likely to demand an acceptable degree of autonomy or room to move as well as the right to contribute to the overall objective setting process. Once again industry has the choice of implementing systems that meet human and social needs as well as technological and business requirements, rather than placing all the emphasis on the latter.

It is evident that many skills have been and will be made redundant by new technology. Such is mankind's identity with work, many people are likely to experience a feeling of society's rejection of their skills and of the contribution they have made and which has provided a social identification for them over many years. Some workers may fear loss of respect or of status or even of employment itself when alternative ways of meeting society's needs are found and implemented. The introduction of technology into production processes has long been a focus of conflict.

An example of de-skilling in the NHS is illustrated by the displacement of the traditional skills of the practical chemist in both the pharmacy and the clinical chemistry laboratory. At the birth of the NHS pharmacists were still to be found concocting various creams, ointments, potions and medicines from component ingredients. Today the 'finished goods' are largely bought-in and pharmacists now place a strong emphasis on advising their medical colleagues on the use and effects of prescribed drugs—they may attend ward rounds for this purpose—and in monitoring drug metabolism in the patient; thus manual (programmed) skills have been substantially replaced by discretionary ones. Some clinical chemistry workers have largely abandoned the glass burette and volumetric pipette for complex automatic chemical analysers which frequently use quite different chemical reactions than were employed in manual analysis. Indeed, skills acquired in operating andmaintaining early analysers of the 1960s and 1970s have already been displaced by yet more complex and sophisticated instruments of the 1980s. This process is likely to continue. As new technology becomes ever more widely applicable to medicine many more occupational skills could be threatened and will require to undergo metamorphosis if some workers are to avoid loss of employment or, at least, reduced job satisfaction.

Changes we have described have an important bearing upon staff selection, recruitment and training. The need now is for flexibility and the acquisition of basic but highly portable skills rather than those specific techniques which characterized the apprenticeship training model. Because in older times one's occupation and craft were believed not to change substantially, skills learned during an apprenticeship would effectively support the craftsman throughout his working life. This model is inadequate for the science-based professions. If skill displacement is to result in re-skilling and role development, as it has done already for some NHS workers, then training and retraining must become an involuntary feature of organisational activity, the cost becoming an overhead of the effective use and implementation of advancing technology.

Since this applies both to knowledge as well as to skills acquisition, many health professions are moving 'up-market' for their recruits, seeking higher educational attainment with wider employment applicability than was deemed necessary before. In the light of such developments, graduate-only entry does not now seem to us an unjustifiable objective for health care professions provided that the discretionary element of their work remains high.

Of course, there are some industrial processes that have caused job function to develop in the opposite direction where the workers are merely de-skilled and the result is a menial and soul-destroying occupation. For example, Rosenbrook has suggested that few workers would object to a robot being used for unpleasant tasks such as paint spraying in confined spaces. But to use a robot to perform a 'skilled' task such as, for example, welding, in pleasant circumstances where the welder could match the performance of the robot, but where the ex-welder is reduced to feeding the robot with fresh work at the completion of each job, is both demeaning and unnecessary. In these circumstances work functions could be reversed to allow the welder to continue to use his skill and the robot to feed in new work when required. However, such work may eventually become totally automated and we face the prospect of whole occupational groups or major parts of them becoming redundant.

Redundancy

The third problem associated with new technology is that it may facilitate staff redundancy, although its track record thus far has not wholly supported this genuine fear amongst NHS workers. The dumping of workers whose skills are no longer required or whose role is no longer compatible with changing management requirements is a shameful waste of human resources. This ought not to occur except by mutual consent. Flexibility should be shown by both the employer and the employee in negotiating either a new employment contract or a redundancy arrangement. Thurley has called for a new range of employment contracts protecting employment but not job security and thereby eliminating waste by the utilization of the potential of people for a variety of jobs during their careers. In this, the reward system of an organisation would need to include worker development as flexibility would become a key characteristic of the new high-tech workers. This is a far cry from the immediate post-war trade union dominated industrial model which led to many demarcation disputes in the UK, if not abroad. It may also serve as a warning to those who currently advocate too high a degree of specialization in job function. Such a commitment to each satisfactory employee would raise morale and facilitate technological progress by the elimination of uncertainty and the maximization of co-operation. Some health authorities already operate a tentative policy in this direction. However, many workers remain fearful that automation, new technology and computers will be used as tools of economic displacement and will be deployed preferentially to human resources in an attempt to reduce the labour-intensive high costs of the NHS.

Future Employment Levels

This is a convenient point at which to examine the evidence as to the likely effects of introducing new technology into the health services. Most, but by no means all, of this technology is computer-based. That is to say a computer, or a microprocessor, is incorporated into a machine or instrument in such a way as to render some human tasks, whether manual, clerical or administrative, unnecessary. As computers are also expected to become increasingly useful in the area of decision-making the breadth of this influence on working practices is potentially very wide. Some writers have predicted that the nature of work itself will be catastrophically changed. Clearly some analytical tools are needed with which to identify and assess the expected changes.

Rajan and Cooke propose a model for the examination of the effects on employment of information technology in the financial service industry. While their model lacks universal applicability it may nevertheless have relevance in other service industries such as theNHS. Banking employment has continued to rise in spite of 25 years of investment in automation and computers. Rajan and Cooke identify a number of factors that influence employment, some of which are capable of moderating adverse effects on employment and others that might accelerate them. These are economic, social and organisational factors. Below, we endeavour to take their model and apply it to the analysis of the likely effect of this technology on employment in the NHS. In the health services generally there has been some investment in new technology, arguably of a broader and different kind from that of banking. While this may have led to some occupational re-skilling, employment levels in health care since 1948 have also continued to rise, particularly in the professions supplementary to medicine. It is mainly these professions which have borne the brunt of the introduction of new technology.

Of course, employment levels are determined by many factors of which new technology is but one. However, one factor in the NHS which is in common with banking is the continual rise in the amount of work undertaken. In the health service there has been a phenomenal increase in, for example, the work of the medical laboratories, the pharmacy and in clinical activities of all kinds. The effect of the steady reduction in the numbers of hospital beds brought about by faster postoperative rehabilitation probably outweighs any impact that labour saving technology has made.

Economic Moderators

The economic moderators that characterize health care centre on the steady growth in demand, and as Culyer has put it, 'the utilization of health services has, on almost every indicator, increased continually since the Second World War'. The more efficient the system becomes at meeting needs, the more needs may be met. In the present context, demand, as indicated by, say, the length of hospital waiting lists (and waiting time) has not been satiated by any means, including new technology. In health care new technology has usually required the acquisition of new skills, or new employees, but the overall number of posts has continued to increase. Where individual worker productivity has risen it has quickly become saturated by increased client demand.

By considering the demand side as well as the supply it is evident that the relationship between new technology and unemployment in health care is far from a simplistic one.

As it appears with banking, new technology has itself created the possibility of new services in health care and stimulated demand. Renal dialysis, bone marrow cancer treatments, and transplant technology generally, are examples of this phenomenon. Neither should this or any other treatment be reviewed solely as a clinical activity. For example, the use of many new drugs associated with these treatments requires monitoring by measuring the blood level of the drug, or its metabolite, in the circulation of the recipient. Special patient monitoring and follow-up are required. Various 'function' tests will be conducted by paramedical staff. Special physiotherapy, perhaps counselling and rehabilitation, may be requested. These are some of the knock-on effects of the technology which permits these new treatments and which themselves stimulate demand.

Because all such treatment is necessarily administered on an individual basis, expansion in the service is likely to require some additional trained staff whose work may be made more effective by new technology rather than be entirely replaced by it. The principal economic factor in the implementation of new technology is Exchequer funding. As we have seen, capital monies are largely divided between building and equipment which will include new technology. Therefore, the funding of technological innovation will largely depend upon the relative demands for new buildings and repairs on existing ones. Where shortage of capital monies gives rise to local income generation by selling services—for example occupational health services or executive health screens—this is deemed likely to result in a positive influence on both staffing levels and equipment utilization. The persistence of lengthy waiting lists in the NHS together with the virtual absence of these in the private health sector indicates that demand in this 'private' market is relatively low at the prevailing price. Therefore, any increase in efficiency in the NHS is likely to stimulate demand further. The recognition and development of consumer awareness by means of Health Maintenance Schemes, Good Practice Allowances for GPs, or by generally raising public expectations will have a similar effect.

Social Moderators

Social factors moderating the impact of new technology are also varied. Rajan and Cooke point to the effects of legislation such as the Employment Protection (Consolidation) Act 1978, which offers some means of job security, and the Health and Safety legislation. Although of uncertain status, to these we would add the Whitley Council Conditions of Service which may yet be instrumental in moderating occupational changes given positive efforts by the trade unions to negotiate successfully new technology and/or natural wastage agreements. The current state and influence of the NHS trade unions is itself a further moderation. For example, the unions may be able to establish with management agreed working practices with new equipment such as the maximum continuous working periods for VDU operators which we believe to be a desirable parameter to define at the present time.

Unlike the experience of banks and building societies where a significant number of customers still prefer personal service to using an automatic cash dispenser or service till, the NHS patient has little need at present to make such a choice. However, we may in future experience the reality of consumer preference in this respect with the emergence of direct patient interrogation by computer. Several systems have been successfully developed and are in regular, though limited, use at various centres in the UK. They are generally specific to particular symptoms and diagnostic areas such as abdominal pain or specific problems such as alcoholism. In these systems the patient sits alone with the computer and responds to questions displayed on the screen by pressing one of four buttons to answer 'yes', 'no', 'don't know' or 'don't understand'. The counterpart for the clinician is the 'expert system' which may be interrogated interactively by the doctor to obtain probable diagnoses from signs, symptoms, history and test results fed in by the enquirer. Experience has already shown that user resistance, amongst other things, is likely to play some moderating part in the introduction of these facilities.

Ultimately we believe that the operation of consumer choice will mean that patients will opt for the approach to diagnosis and treatment that best meets their needs. In the majority of cases this will favour strategies that are technically and economically efficient. One important facet of computer/client interaction is that a computer need never be rude, aggressive or overbearing to any patient; it need never be forgetful in questioning or judgemental in response. A computer can be programmed to be infinitely patient and to give straight and uncomplicated replies. Furthermore it is feasible to combine medical 'expert systems' with direct client interrogation facilities to provide commercial 'do-it-yourself diagnostic kits for home use. Our guess is that such a development would be most likely to raise further the public consciousness of health issues and lower the threshold at which demand is made on the professional health services.

Orgnizational Moderators

Organisational moderators relate both to policy and to its likely effect upon staff. This in turn relates mainly to an organisation's propensity to change and the manner in which that change occurs. Investment in new technology may also mean a loss of return on previous investment in people and in older technology and the 'wasting' of much experience through *de facto* occupational redundancy. Since staff are usually regarded as the most important investment a company can make, most organisations may be expected to consider ways of optimizing the return on this and indeed on all their investments including new technology.

With respect to the implementation of change, the statement by Griffiths that The effectiveness of the NHS depends on the staff it employs, and a better run service will mean a more satisfied customer, a happier working environment and a more satisfied staff, is the traditional and legitimate view of most successful organisations including the NHS. The sub-culture maintained by such an attitude is a valuable source of motivation and most organisations may be expected to seek to preserve, enhance and make use of it during any change brought about by the introduction of new technology. A further point implied by Rajan and Cooke is that where there exists a multiplicity of tasks associated with the operation of an enterprise the automation of one aspect of a task, as in the case of, say, a word processor, may have little impact on overall staffing levels, especially where the machine can be used more to improve the quality of the production of service than to speed production.

Until fairly recently many computer applications have evolved following local (district) design and development in collaboration with computer companies. This has not usually threatened local staffing levels. Now the control and/or ownership of substantial computer systems appears to be passing to Regional Health Authorities, and with this the realization that there are as yet no staffing norms associated with any new technology. It may be expected that endeavours will be made to correct this omission in the near future.

Accelerating Factors

As with financial institutions it appears that in the health sector, also, growth and demand have been the chief moderator of staffing levels in the face of new technology. We believe it is the current attempt by central government to regulate demand that may constitute a departure from the pattern established since 1948 and accelerate the technological impact on employment. The combination of tight financial controls, together with strong directives from the centre, both to increase economic efficiency and to implement new and wide-ranging computer-based information systems, such as the Korner data requirements. may be significant in this respect and help to establish a tendency to maximize staff savings from increased productivity. Management information is most economically gathered as a by-product of normal activity and many special manual and computer systems at present solely used for the collection of Korner data are likely to have short and uneconomic life cycles. The continuing emphasis on community networks linking hospitals, community health centres and general practitioners is growing and may be expected to expedite the deployment and integration of computer systems and related technology generally.

We may yet see in the health service a phenomenon equivalent to the deliberate and centrally (government) engineered 'shake-out' that occurred in British industry in the early eighties. Then many firms were forced to address resolutely the problem of overmanning in order to survive and those who failed to do this were destroyed. We recognize that such a thought is alien and repugnant to most workers in the caring professions who have come to regard their personal nurturing and caring ethos to be synonymous with that of their employing organisation. Neither are purely commercial equations naively applicable to health care since by definition and by common consent this is a labour-intensive activity. However, there is no reason we can find to condone genuine inefficiency and, as opportunities present, given the influence of the many moderating and accelerating factors involved, we expect to see, in due course, various substitutions and new strategies, including the use of new technology in order to improve economic efficiency and effectiveness in the service. In this context we would expect employment levels in some NHS occupations to fall.

Organisation Development

So far we have discussed some of the factors that may be expected to influence staffing strategy in the NHS. In spite of today's preoccupation with technological development we remain firmly of the opinion that any organisation's most important and valuable asset is its staff. It is because of new technology, changes in the labour market and of economic factors generally that our most pressing problems within organisations concern change. By this we mean, for example, changes in job functions, professional groupings and alignments, goal affinities and skill requirements. In particular, the possibility of non-incremental change is exacerbated by new technology within both many organisations and their various environments. Union-management agreements that are assumed to have been set in stone now require revision. By the same token the professional ethos with its acquired 'immunities' from critical examination has, until recently, remained unchallenged. Now, exposed by the pressure for change, many professional rules appear to support restrictive practices even though they may have originated to protect clients and the general public.

The dilemma for authority has always been the source of its legitimacy. If an organisation does not act by virtue of absolute power—a dangerous strategy to adopt in a democracy—it must rely on a variety of persuasive and logical reasons aimed at obtaining compliance with its wishes and plans. In most cases this will involve obtaining a majority agreement or consensus of opinion of members of that organisation.

In a complex coalescence of professional and occupational groups such as comprise the National Health Service the ability to enforce worker compliance regardless of their resistance is extremely limited and is only likely to operate in the short term, if at all. Moreover, recognition of legitimate authority, as in Weber's Rational Legal ideal type is often given first to a worker's profession, professional organisation or trade union. Alternatively, personal value systems regarding appropriate patient care may command more loyalty from workers and exhibit greater institutional effect than organisational edicts that are handed down from management. In these circumstances many workers may find ways of circumventing an edict thus effectively demonstrating that the rational legal authority is incompletely legitimized.

We recognize that there will always be differences of opinion between workers and that the value of conflict in organisations is far from being always negative. However, the question we are addressing is how are we to achieve and control change in an organisation as complex as the NHS as opposed to a much simpler one such as a national grocery chain? The answer to this is itself complicated. In part the answer lies in obtaining the agreement of all, or at least a majority, of staff to identify with, implement and maintain new working practices, workload norms and organisational changes that will make our practice of health care more effective. By involving staff at the beginning of the change exercise rather than confronting them with a ready-made decision and action plan, the organisation increases its chances of long-term success. Conflicts of values may be openly discussed and uncertainties of outcome, a source of much stress and resistance to change, may be placed in the hands of those directly affected and hence to some extent may become self-determining. It is this consensual strategy which forms one of the distinguishing features of organisation development. The section on management training, where we discussed the need for trainers to work 'alongside' individuals or groups and assist them to solve current rather than idealized problems.

Williams defines organisation development (OD) as a term whichis applied to certain types of planned efforts at bringing about organisational change. We need not be concerned here to find a more elaborate definition since we wish to avoid categorization and the possible exclusion of otherwise helpful knowledge and methodology. What is clear is that OD addresses the problems of organisational change by working inside the organisation, tapping into the ideas, experience and energies of its constituent workers individually, or in groups, to effect agreed changes that are mutually beneficial. For this an OD specialist is usually employed. Such specialists frequently bear the title of management consultant. This is a pity, for in our view it does nothing to differentiate them from any other kind of management 'expert'.

Traditionally, management experts in general have employed a diagnosis and prescription technique, often known as 'hit and run'. A management consultant would typically use a 'Top Down' approach looking at organisational structure, business policy, staffing and outputs. A prescriptive solution to the problem would be tendered (together with a hefty invoice for services rendered) and the organisation left to implement a *de facto,* management-imposed change as best it could. When things went wrong one could always blame the consultant, as many blamed McKinsey and Co. in 1974.

Other consultants might take a more analytical 'Bottom Up' approach and spend time analysing working practice through Method Study and Work Measurement. Before the solution is presented there may be a great deal of discussion with relevant workers but ownership of the problem and of the change strategy is perceived to be with the management consultant. As a consquence, the solution, or alternative solutions, when announced, are frequently ascribed with a parental ethos and although the consultant may continue to be present during implementation, that support is necessarily limited and ownership of the prescription is never effectively transferred. No consultant can continue supporting an organisation indefinitely and so the OD approach aims never to remove ownership of a problem from the organisation. Instead it provides help and expertise and facilitative skill in assisting the workers themselves to identify and solve their own problems and to bring about their own organisational change. This involves the OD worker in the recognition of all salient factors that go to make up the organisation's culture, a willingness to listen to all points of view, an ability to spot where the proffered solutions are unlikely to work and to recognize when genuine progress is being made. At the same time the OD worker must never personally take responsibility for either the problem or for finding the solution (or credit for the accepted solution) and must know when it is appropriate to commence withdrawing support.

An OD worker, then, will adopt a flexible style which will not be that of an expert delivering judgement nor of a teacher imparting knowledge but will be that of a facilitator enabling the clients to diagnose their problems before searching for solutions and to consider alternatives before choosing a preferred solution. It follows that all individuals and groups that have a vested interest in the addressed problem that can affect the outcome of any solution must be involved from the outset.

It could be argued that this approach reduces management to the status merely of an interested party and effectively removes its 'right to manage'. In fact it does nothing of the kind. In our view this is not a helpful way of viewing OD. The rights of management are best considered in parallel with its responsibilities and are legitimized to a great extent as those responsibilities are met. The responsibilities we have in mind include the process of consultation, communication and commitment to staff. Since coercion is likely always to provoke resistance the OD strategy would seem to be a useful initial approach to a wide variety of problems, some of which might be tackled in-house particularly if staff have had previous OD experience. The more an organisation can learn to solve its own problems the better for all its members and the less expense is incurred in employing consultants.

Where total resistance to change is encountered, however, management have a number of legal options but these should be carefully evaluated before use. In our view the characteristics of strong management are confidence, leadership and a willingness to listen. Those of weak management are aggressiveness towards staff and an inability to be even-handed, which leads to unbalanced or extreme decisions which require strong sanctions to impose and maintain.

Lewin, in his field force theory put forward a model of organisational change based upon three steps.

1. Unfreezing the Current Situation's Controlling Forces

These include current conceptions, working practices or ideological beliefs. For this, workers may be placed in learning situations such as being exposed to new technology job methodologies in order to create dissatisfaction with the existing situation and thus create a desire for change. In practice this does not always work and more coercive techniques have been employed, particularly where change is required rapidly. The threat of redundancy and the acquaintance of staff with the fact of managerial power, say, for example, to change unilaterally contracts of employment, may 'unfreeze' attitudes and bring agreement that change is after all possible. However, this holds within it thedangers of long-term remembered pain by the workforce and entrenched dissatisfaction.

2. Finding and Implementing Change

Only when the unfreezing is complete is it worth embarking on the quest for change and involving workers in a search for preferred alternatives which satisfy the aspirations of all parties. This serves to emphasize that a change agent or OD worker is required to be invited to assist staff in their quest and not to be unilaterally imposed as the agent of management to browbeat workers into submission. However, where Stage 1 does not call for such measures the OD worker can have a valuable part to play. For example, where problems arise with inappropriate role perceptions between different groups of co-workers the OD worker will use his or her skills to bring such groups together, help them to communicate effectively and facilitate new patterns of work and behaviour.

3. Refreezing the New Situation's Controlling Forces

When change is agreed its implementation needs to be established by positive reinforcement. This may take the form of rewards inherent in the new system of work and it is important to recognize that change decisions are unlikely to stick if no such rewards are forthcoming. For example, some of the spectacular failures of some medical computer systems may be attributable to just this lack of reward. In any case steps need to be taken to refreeze the forces maintaining the new situation, remembering that transient behavioural change may be analagous to a remission rather than a cure. This further emphasizes the need for the OD worker to support each project until all stages are complete, i.e. not only assisting with diagnosis and treatment but with convalescence as well.

There are several ways in which different OD strategies may be classified depending upon their context and approach. These are summarized broadly by Williams as:

Team development

Inter-group development

Total organisation development

Improving the match between people and jobs

Improving the match between organisations and their environment.

OD And The NHS

Recently the NHS Training Authority stated:

'Change is endemic in most large organisations and the NHS is no exception. Innovations in medical care, shifting priorities, new organisation structures, revised funding levels and varying public expectations, are just a few of the changes which health service managers are currently having to consider.

'In 1985 the National Health Service Training Authority set up the Change Management Consultancy Programme, and began to recruit a cadre of OD workers, to be known as

Change Management Consultants, drawn from a variety of backgrounds within the NHS, and to train them as part of the Programme to work with client authorities. 'Change Management Consultants help their clients to develop and 'own' their own solutions to problems. They assist in defining change issues, in working out how to tackle them and in seeing them through to conclusion. They also aim to leave the client organisation with an enhanced ability to handle change in the future. The style of the Programme focuses much attention on behavioural aspects of each project as well as calling for diagnostic, problem solving facilitating and counselling skills.'

In this way the ideas of OD are being appropriated to pursue the policy of the NHS Training Authority in order that:

1. The ownership of management development, which includes the ability to manage change, remains a local responsibility with appropriate support.
2. Management development be regarded as a comprehensive and continuous process for all rather than be characterized by sporadic episodes of training for a privileged few.

It is easy to think that OD presents an infallible guide to the way forward with respect to organisational change. But it is a major and effective approach to be used wherever appropriate and particularly where consensus may be difficult, but highly desirable, to attain.

4

Dimensions of Public Health Research, Hospital Management Policy and Medical Ethics

CASE STUDY: MANAGER AND LAW IN U.K. HOSPITALS

The legal system in England and Wales originates from Norman times when the Norman Kings established the centre of the legal system in London. The system of Assize Courts outside London was established by Henry II, who took judges with him in his processions around the country to deliberate on local disputes. The British legal system, or variations of it, has since been established around the world due to its exportation with the British Empire and throughout the Commonwealth—the pomp of bewigged judges and jury-made decisions lives on. Managers in the health care professions are most likely to need a knowledge of civil rather than criminal law, particularly of the areas of employment and contract law. As can be seen, there is a system of appeals against lower court decisions to higher level courts. For managers in health care it is the industrial tribunals and their appellate court in the Queen's Bench Division, the EAT (Employment Appeals Tribunal), as well as, possibly, the Commercial Court, which are likely to be the most important and with which they are most likely to become involved. The decisions of the highest courts bind the lower ones and the system of judge-made precedents is a unique feature of the English legal system and establishes what is known as the Common Law. The other major source of law is Statute Law which is established by Acts of Parliament or Statutory Instruments, largely through government-inspired legislation or, since 1971 and our membership of the European Community, through EEC Directives.

EMPOLYMENT LAW

Common law governs the contract of employment. It need not be written down but in practice it should be, although an oral contract is binding. It governs the formation of the contract, its express and implied terms, and matters arising during the course of the employment, e.g. confidentiality of information gained through the employment, termination of the contract and post-termination restrictions such as the non-disclosure of confidential information. These common law rights are only applicable to employees, not independent contractors or the self-employed as the employment contract is a contract of service, not one to provide a service.

Statute law is superimposed, grafted onto, the common law, its purpose being to regulate the employment relationship and prevent inequality. The statutes of which managers need knowledge cover the individual rights of employees to be given written particulars of the main terms and conditions of employment, equal pay and equal opportunity for both males and females and all racial groups, maternity rights, the right not to be unfairly dismissed and redundancy payment rights. These statutory rights provide a legal minimum 'floor of rights' which would override any less generous terms or conditions in an employment contract.

Obviously, employers can be more generous if they wish to be, for example the Whitley Council redundancy pay conditions, which are more generous than the statutory minimum.

The Legal Obligations in the Employment Relationship

1. The first aspect of the contract of employment that needs to be emphasized is its personal nature. Duties and obligations apply to both the employer and employee and the employment contract is thus given special treatment by the courts in that, unlike a commercial contract, it is rare for either side to be compelled to carry out any specific clause of the contract. This does occasionally happen as when an injunction can be granted against an employee forbidding the disclosure of confidential information or when, very rarely, an employer is ordered to re-employ the employee, but it is far more usual for the tribunal's or courts' remedy to take the form of damages for breach of contract.

2. There are various implied duties of the employer:

(a) Mutual respect. Employers have a legal duty to treat employees with due respect and consideration, being mindful of their duties and problems; for example, the employer has a duty to train and supervise new and probationary staff properly and to provide safe equipment and a healthy environment in which to carry out the work.

(b) To provide work. The very nature of an employment contract is that a person is employed and remunerated for some mental or physical labour. An employer is, though, under no legal obligation to provide work unless it adversely affects an employee's actual or potential earnings, or unless the employee is an apprentice in training, but it would obviously be a foolish, or a particularly philanthropic, employer who paid staff for doing no work.

(c) To pay wages/remuneration when no work is available. An employer is obliged to pay employees who are available for work even when there is none, unless he has written an express term into the contract giving him the right to lay people off without pay. The State guarantees to provide 5 days' pay in any one quarter for anyone laid off in this way.

(d) To indemnify. The employer must meet any expenses reasonably and properly incurred by an employee in the course of his employment, but this would not apply to expenses which are not reasonably and properly incurred, such as parking fines.

(e) References. There is no legal obligation on an employer to provide references for employees. It is far wiser not to give a reference than to give a false one, as if an employee is untruthfully commended, the next employer could take action against the former employer for damages due to deceit/misrepresentation. In an unfair dismissal case, the giving of a glowing reference for someone in order to get rid of him can rebound and, therefore, the best advice is never to say things about an employee that are untrue.

(f) To ensure the employee's safety. There is a duty of reasonable care on an employer in both common law and statute law. Any breach can, therefore, lead to a two-fold action as the purpose of common law is to compensate for injuries incurred as a result of an employer's negligence, and the purpose of the statute law is accident prevention, enforced by criminal penalties against the employer. Therefore, in the case of an accident to an employee at work, one could be awarded compensation under common law and damages under statute law.

3. The duty of care of employers. This duty has three main elements, which impose a personal obligation on an employer which cannot be delegated. These elements are a duty to provide:

(a) Plant and appliances which are reasonably safe to work.

(b) A system of work which must be safe in areas such as layout, training, supervision and protective clothing.

(c) Fellow employees must be reasonably competent. Higher standards of care are placed on employers when dealing with inexperienced employees or those whose English is poor and so greater precautions must be taken in these situations. If an employer is found to have been negligent in any of these areas, he can be held to be vicariously liable for the acts of his employees. The employer's normal defences against negligence actions are to deny negligence, transfer blame to the employees, or claim contributory negligence. Under the Unfair Contract Terms Act 1977, an employer cannot seek to exclude liability for death and personal injury by putting up a notice to that effect. Where an employee brings an action for negligence or nuisance for a breach of the employer's statutory duty involving personal injury, this must be brought within three years from the date when the injury occurred or the date when the claimant had knowledge of the injury.

4. There are various implied obligations of the employee.

(a) Duty of fidelity to work honestly and in good faith.

(b) To obey all lawful and reasonable orders.

(c) To perform work competently, using reasonable skill and care.

(d) Not to accept secret bribes, commissions or gifts.

(e) Not to disclose confidential information to an unauthorized person for the employee's own purpose, both during and after termination, except when obliged by law to do so.

(f) Under the Patents Act 1977 8.39 any invention which an employee might create as a result of his normal duties or specific assignments and which might reasonably result from these duties or because of his obligation to further the business interests of his employer, would lead to the invention belonging to the employer. In any other situation the right to patent the invention would belong to the employee. If the employee felt an invention had been of outstanding benefit to his employer and he had not been adequately rewarded for it he could apply to the Patents Court for compensation to be paid by his employer.

(g) Not to act in any manner which is inconsistent with the duty of fidelity.

(h) To indemnify the employer if, by the employee's negligence a third party is injured.

(i) To compensate the employer for any loss suffered resulting from a breach of contractual obligations.

The Drafting and Revision of Contracts of Employment

The contract of employment is the key source document in the employment relationship and the health care manager and the employing authority should use it to provide maximum flexibility for the location of the staffs employment and the duties to be carried out by each member of staff, as well as achieving certainty for the rights and obligations of both parties to the employment contract. Ideally, it should be a fluid and evolving document, reflecting changing organisational needs and requirements and increasing or decreasing areas of responsibility and specialization of the individual employee. It is important that it does not become a static or archaic document and that it is regularly reviewed, the major areas to be concerned with in drafting and revision being:

1. Ensuring the correct date of the commencement of duties. Since many of the rights of employees, examined later in this study, are time-related, it is important that this date is accurate. Also, district health authorities are not automatically held to be associated employers and, therefore, it is important that this is explicitly stated to ensure continuity of service between one authority and another in the NHS.

2. Reference should be made to the job title and the general job duties and explicit reference should be made to the job description which, as has already been recommended should be comprehensive and regularly updated. The major point about the job description from the employment law viewpoint is that it should provide as much management flexibility as possible in order to prevent claims for constructive dismissal from employees.

3. The place of work should be stated and if this could be at a variety of sites or locations, then this must be explicitly stated.

4. Hours of work and overtime rates, if they apply, should be explicitly stated.

5. Remuneration:

(a) The sum, or where it may be found, i.e. the appropriate salary scale in the standard terms and conditions of service.

(b) The method of payment—whether by cash, cheque or credit transfer, weekly or monthly, and the date on which payment will be made.

(c) Car allowance—explicitly stating who pays for repairs, road tax, petrol and insurance or, again, referring to the relevant terms and conditions.

(d) Bonuses and any other performance-linked payments.

6. Exclusivity of services. Reference is often made to the employer's right to vet any other work done by an employee and to be directly reimbursed for it, or to prevent an employee doing it if it is felt to interfere with the employee's primary full-time employment. Other restrictions could relate to non-disclosure of confidential information, restrictions on future employment by rival companies, and the employer's right to the copyright of inventions of employees.

7. Holidays. Their length and when they have to be taken should be stated as well as the rights of employees to carry them over from year to year, or to have to accept payment in lieu if no such right exists.

8. Expenses. What expenses are allowable and at what rates.

9. Sick pay. The period of entitlement, whether contractual or discretionary, and the rules governing notification of illness, absence, and the medical evidence required—when to telephone, self-certification, medical certification.

10. Other benefits given by the authority in excess of the statutory provision.

11. Grievance and disputes procedure. The method of raising a complaint or grievance should be stated as well as the method of disciplinary action. Ideally, there should be at least one verbal warning, a written warning, clearly stated and recorded, and a final written warning, but the rights should be clearly reserved in the contract to go direct to the final written warning stage and to dismiss immediately, without warning, for gross misconduct.

12. Notice of termination. The period on either side should be clearly stated and this must be at least the statutory minimum of under 2 years' service, 1 week's notice, and from 2-12 years, 1 week plus 1 week for each year of service up to a maximum of 12 weeks. Any probationary period of service should be clearly referred to, and the discretion to pay salary in lieu of notice should be reserved.

It is thus clear that there are a great many topics which should be clearly covered in the employment contract and, therefore, in order to keep the contract document itself reasonably short, it is wise to put all the elaborate procedures such as Statutory Sick Pay, examples of gross misconduct, and specific Whitley terms and conditions relating to the particular contract, in a separate document to which the employee can make reference. It is probably true to say that there is a greater onus of care in the discharge of contractual terms and conditions placed on health authorities and health care managers, as public employees, than might apply to a private sector company which certainly seems to be borne out in the case of Irani v. Southampton and S.W. Hants Health Authority (1985) where an injunction to perform the contract was upheld against the Authority for not carrying out the disciplinary procedure laid down in the employment contract. This emphasizes the need to keep terms and conditions updated and to change them when they become outdated.

Changing the Employment Contract

As the employment contract is formed by mutual agreement over terms and conditions of service, any change or variation must be mutual unless the employee's agreement to the changes have already been expressed in the original contract, for example, by his agreeing to be employed, say, anywhere in the district, or to work any amount of overtime demanded. Obviously, the more open the wording of the original terms and conditions of a contract, the less problems the employer will have in changing it and the employee will have far greater problems in rejecting changes. If an employee's agreement to changes cannot be inferred from the contract, then the employer will have to seek the agreement of the employee to changes, impose it on him, or back down from trying to introduce changes. If the change is unilaterally imposed, then the employee would either have to accept it, or resign and claim constructive dismissal on the grounds that the employer had repudiated a material and fundamental term of the contract relating to pay, hours or status. This would involve taking the employer to an industrial tribunal. The tribunal would apply the test of reasonableness to the claim—if the contract change was held to be fair, then the employee's claim would be dismissed, if it was held to be unfair, then compensation would be awarded.

If the employee refused to accept the changes and did not resign, the employer would have to dismiss him. This could lead to a claim for unfair dismissal and/or a redundancy payment claim. Employers are often faced with these difficulties over changing contracts when they are either trying to cut costs or restructure their organisations to make them more efficient. It is open to the employer to argue that the breach of contract was reasonable in all the circumstances because of business needs so that the dismissal was not unfair, or that suitable alternative employment had been offered to the employee so that, by rejecting it, he had lost his entitlement to redundancy pay. The tribunal members have to apply an objective test of reasonableness, for example 10 minutes' extra travelling time per day might be considered reasonable, but an extra hour unreasonable, due to a re-siting of employment. An employer would be expected to provide graphs and statistics to prove that there were sound business reasons for a change of contract and so long as he can do this he will normally be held to have acted fairly. If an entirely new contract was to be imposed on staff, then notice of termination of the old one would have to be given before issuing the new contracts or revised terms. If the employees accept the proposed changes then this is not required and they can just countersign a letter outlining the changes and stating that 'all other terms and conditions will remain unchanged'.

Unfair Dismissal

The concept of unfair dismissal and the establishment of industrial tribunals, which comprise a legally trained chairman and two lay members, one TUC nominated and one CBI nominated, was initially introduced by Edward Heath's Conservative government in the 1971 Industrial Relations Act. Unfair dismissal claims are currently governed by the 1978 Employment Protection (Consolidation) Act (EPCA) and any employee who feels he has been unfairly dismissed has to hold the status of an employee and not an independent contractor in order to be able to make a claim. If the employee's continuous service commenced before 1 June, 1985 then the qualifying period of service he has to have is one year before a claim for unfair dismissal can be brought. Anyone employed on or after 1 June, 1985 has to have 2 years' continuous service before being able to make such a claim. The legislation only applies to those who normally work in Great Britain and the claim must be presented within 3 months of the effective date of termination. The employee must not be over the normal retirement age applicable in the employer's business, or the statutory retirement age. An employee would also, obviously, be unable to make a claim if he had expressly waived his rights to do so in a specific term of the contract.

Effective Date of Termination

This will differ according to the terms of the dismissal. If the contractual period of notice, e.g. 1 month, is given, then the normal date of termination would be the end of the notice period. If the employee was on a fixed term contract then the effective date of termination would be the end of the contract term. However, an employer could ask an employee to leave immediately and pay him his due salary in lieu of the notice as compensation. If that was done, then the effective date of termination would be the last day the employee worked and the employee would get his salary, in lieu of notice, free of income tax, so it would be advantageous both to him, as well as to the employer. If the employer decided to pay him over the notice period but asked him to stay at home and not attend for work then the last day of the contract would be the end of the notice period.

Dismissal

Three situations satisfy dismissal in law—direct employer termination, expiry of a fixed-term contract without renewal, and constructive dismissal. Resignation by an employee, his leaving by mutual agreement, or a supervening event leading to the termination of a contract, such as a person being in jail for over a year, or a serious long-term illness, do not rank as dismissals.

For a dismissal to be fair, an employer has to prove

that an employee has been dismissed for an 'admissible' reason. This would be misconduct, poor performance—an employee who after counselling cannot perform the duties of the joh—long-term ill health, redundancy—either through moving of the business or because the needs of a business for a particular employee's skills have ceased or diminished—or where continued employment would result in a breach of a statute, e.g. an employee holding no work permit when one is required or an employee who loses his driving licence and has to drive in order to do his job properly, or 'some other substantial reason', e.g. a breakdown in customer relations leading to customer pressure to dismiss the employee, or a genuine business reorganisation. The non-admission of some earlier criminal offence prior to employment might also be held to be fair grounds for dismissal so long as it was not held to be a 'spent' conviction under the 1974 Rehabilitation of Offenders Act. An employee can be instantly dismissed, without warning, for gross misconduct, which would normally be held to be theft, violent behaviour or breach of contract.

An employer has to bring his reason for dismissal into one of the categories outlined above, in order for a dismissal to be held to be fair if an employee decided to bring a claim for unfair dismissal at an industrial tribunal. The tribunal has to be happy that the admissible reason was 'fair in all the circumstances at the time the employer dismissed and having regard to the size of the company and its resources'. Therefore, high standards would be expected of a health authority and its managers but as long as any health authority ensures that its managers are knowledgeable about the information given in this study then no problems should arise. The tribunal would also take account of the way the authority and its managers went about the dismissal, that the necessary warnings were properly given, the disputes procedure followed and that adequate consultation took place before redundancies, if they were carried out. In applying the general fairness test to the admissible reasons the industrial tribunal would use the following criteria:

1. Gross misconduct. It could be held to be fair to dismiss the employee without any warning, but the manager's best approach svould probably be to suspend an employee suspected of theft or violent behaviour on full pay, until full investigations into the incident have been satisfactorily completed, particularly if there is any doubt. This should include giving the employee sufficient detail about the charges against him, for him to provide an adequate defence to the charges at a formal interview before final dismissal takes place. If someone is charged by the police the employer must still carry out his own investigations and decide whether 'on balance of probabilities' he committed the crime. This would be held to be a reasonable test and his guilt would not be expected to be proved 'beyond reasonable doubt'. Again, the procedure should be to suspend, investigate and give the employee the chance to put his side of the case, before deciding whether the offence had been committed and taking action.
2. Minor misconduct. If the employee was a poor performer or a poor timekeeper, then the test of fairness would be whether the disciplinary procedure had been properly carried out. This, according to the ACAS code should consist of a first verbal warning which could be informal or formal, a first written warning and a second written warning. Before issuing a warning the employer could make sure he has confronted the employee and listened to his side of the case—if the employer does not agree with it, he

should go ahead with issuing the warning. The first warning given usually refers to the next stage of the disciplinary procedure, and the fact that unless specified satisfactory improvements take place, over a specified time period during which the monitoring of performance will take place, then further disciplinary action in line with the established disciplinary procedure will follow. At each stage it would be usual to allow a union representative or fellow-employee to attend the procedure, and it would be usual to allow such attendance at a meeting to formalize the first verbal warning. It is perfectly in order for the disciplinary procedure to allow a jump from the first to the final stage where serious, but not quite gross misconduct has occurred. The procedure should allow the employee a reasonable chance to improve between warnings. Full use should be made of the legislative limitations on employees being allowed to bring claims and certain levels of performance should be expected of employees in their first 18 months' employment which should be written into the training schedule and referred to in the employment contract, to enable a swift and easy parting if the recruitment procedures prove to have failed to recruit a suitable person.

3. Capability. There need to be fair procedures for dealing with incapability and attempts to improve competence by retraining schemes or improved supervision need to be attempted before disciplinary action is embarked on. In the case of long-term illness, it is necessary to ascertain the true medical position, possibly by means of an independent medical examination, before any decision is made to end the company's sickness leave procedures and either offer the employee reasonable alternative employment

or dismiss him. Malingerers or employees with a lot of sickness absence which seemed unjustified would be held to have committed misconduct, even if it was certified absence, and so long as a proper disciplinary procedure was carried out they would be held to be fairly dismissed by an industrial tribunal.

4. Redundancy. There is a need to demonstrate fair selection criteria in deciding whom to make redundant and whether it has been fairly applied. This might be based on a last in first out criterion but it does not have to be, if there is some other laid down policy with specified criteria. These could include: employee's qualifications, flexibility, performance and attendance records. Employees must be warned that redundancy is coming and often the first step is to consult en masse and ask for the requisite number of volunteers. If these are not enough, then the established criteria have to be used for selection. It is advantageous, as noted earlier, for the employee to be given pay in lieu of notice as no tax is payable on such payments. These are often more than the statutory minimum and are tax-free under £25 000.

Redundancy is defined under section 81 of the EPCA as dismissal 'attributable wholly or mainly to the employer ceasing or intending to cease to continue his business for the purposes of which the employee was employed or continuing it in a certain place, and the work of the employee has, or is going to, diminish'. In order to qualify for redundancy, an employee has to have a minimum of 2 years' service, hold a contract of employment, be normally employed in Great Britain, and not be over retirement age. The amount of statutory redundancy pay is calculated on the formula:

½ week's pay for every year of employment between ages 18 and 21

1 week's pay for every year of employment between ages 22 and 40

1 week's pay for every year of employment over age 41.

A maximum of 20 years' service can be taken into account with the maximum amount of weekly pay being £152.

If 10 or more people are to be made redundant, then the rules and provisions of sections 99-107 of the 1975 Employment Protection Act must be followed. Under these, any independent recognized trade union, and the Secretary of State for Employment, have to be informed on Form HR1 of the reasons for redundancy, the numbers involved, the descriptions of the types of employees, the method of their selection, and the proposed procedure for making them redundant. The trade union has to be informed of non-members as well as members. Where 100 or more employees are to be made redundant within a 90-day period, then the notification and consultation procedure must begin at least 90 days before the first person is made redundant. If between 10 and 99 people are to be made redundant within a 30-day period, then the procedure must begin at least 30 days before the first redundancy. If between 1 and 9 staff are to be made redundant within 30 days or less, no specified period is laid down for notification and consultation. Last in, first out, is generally the rule adopted for redundancies, but this can be varied depending on where people are employed as, obviously, an employer will only want to make staff redundant in areas of the organisation where cutbacks are required. If it is impossible to reach agreement with the employees and the union over whom should be made redundant and how, then the employer can be taken to an industrial tribunal by the union, under S. 101 of the 1975 Act, or by the employees, under S. 103. The tribunal will look at whether the statutory procedures have been complied with and, if not, it can award 2 weeks' wages to each employee. An employer can reclaim a 35% rebate on his redundancy payments from the State on Forms RP1 and RP2 but this can be reduced by up to 10% if the notification and consultation procedures are not properly administered, or the HR1 form is not delivered on time. Redundancy pay can be forfeited by employees for striking, an unreasonable refusal of an offer of suitable alternative employment, misconduct during the notice period, or leaving before the end of the notice period without the employer's consent.

Compensation for Unfair Dismissal

Any staff who are held by an industrial tribunal to have been unfairly dismissed are entitled to:

1. A basic award calculated on a sliding scale based on age, length of service and salary. As with redundancy payments the maximum number of years to be taken account of is 20, the maximum for a week's pay is £152 gross and an employee can be compensated on the basis of a week's pay for every year of service under 22, 1 week's pay for every complete year of service between 22 and 41, and 1 week's pay for every complete year of service over 41. Thus, the maximum payment is £4560 under the basic award. The maximum gross pay payable usually increases annually by £10 per year.
2. A compensatory award can be made to cover financial loss, resulting from the unfair dismissal, up to a maximum figure of £8000. This award can cover any loss of net earnings until the tribunal considers the employee will obtain, or has obtained, a new job, and the loss of any perks or contractual benefits. This sum is added to the basic award. The employee is under a duty to take all reasonable steps to find

a new job promptly—he cannot sit and wait for his losses to mount to the £8000 limit and then claim it back. The sum awarded can be reduced if the employee is held to have contributed to his own dismissal.

3. An additional award can be made for failure to comply with an order by the tribunal that an employee should be re-instated or reengaged. Such an order is the first decision a tribunal can adopt, but often employers are unwilling to accept it, and prefer to make this additional award to free themselves of the employee. Such awards have only been made in 5% of the cases brought to industrial tribunals since their establishment, but they mean that the tribunal can award a further 13-26 weeks' pay. With the maximum £152 gross applying, this means an extra sum of £1976-£3952. If the employee was dismissed on the illegal grounds of sex or race, then higher awards of between 26 and 52 weeks' pay can be given, sums of between £3952 and £7904.
4. A special award can be made for closed shop dismissals or union membership/activities dismissals. If re-instatement is sought but not ordered, then 2 years' pay within the range of £10 500-£21 000 can be awarded. If re-instatement is ordered, but not complied with, then 3 years' pay can be awarded up to a current maximum of £15 750 a year, a maximum £47 250.

As long as the various disciplinary procedures outlined in this study are followed, then any dismissal which has to take place is likely to be fair, and any claims by employees for unfair dismissal should be fought, otherwise vituperative employees may deliberately cause problems and threaten to go to an industrial tribunal in the hope of being paid off by a weak or inefficient employer. If an employer knows he has acted incorrectly, but was willing to do so in order to get rid of an inefficient or disruptive employee, then it would obviously be pointless for the employer to fight an unfair dismissal claim as the costs of doing so would probably only add to his final bill. It is always wise to make offers of settlement to aggrieved employees off the record, and to state they are without prejudice, as, if a written offer of settlement is made, this could be produced by the employee at a tribunal hearing to support his case and to increase his award. When a verbal agreement or settlement has been reached with an employee, and he has agreed to waive any claims against the employer in return for a specific monetary settlement, then a letter specifying the terms of settlement should be drawn up. This should state the date of severance, the level of compensation, the compensatory treatment of fringe benefits, pension and reference provision, and that these terms constitute a full and final settlement of any claim, that the details of it must not be disclosed by the employee, and that it is subject to prior ratification by ACAS. The ratification of any settlement by an ACAS official is vital, and all the health authority has to do is to contact ACAS and get one of their officers to speak to the employee, after which he has to sign a COT 3 settlement form waiving his rights to go to an industrial tribunal. If this procedure is not followed, the employee could still re-open the case, and go to an industrial tribunal which would not take account of any previous payment made under a private arrangement that had not been ratified by ACAS, and could, therefore, order further compensation.

Maternity Rights

A major area of employment legislation concerns the rights of female employees who become pregnant. These rights are based on the concept of all the sex discrimination laws which aim to provide women with equal job security with men in line with the stresses and responsibilities of motherhood. The four rights which apply during and after pregnancy relate to:

1. The right to time off work for antenatal care—S. 31 of the 1978 Employment Protection (Consolidation) Act.
2. The right to maternity pay of nine-tenths of a week's pay, less the State maternity allowance for a period of 6 weeks—S. 34.
3. The right to return to work following pregnancy—S. 35.
4. The right not to be unfairly dismissed for any reason linked with pregnancy—S. 60.

The one qualification for these rights is that the female employee must have been employed for 2 years as at the llth week before the expected date of confinement, by that employer, or an associated employer.

Time Off for Antenatal Care

This applies to the second and subsequent attendances and not to thefirst. The first visit is excluded because a woman could keep saying she was attending an antenatal clinic when she was not pregnant and so it is aimed at avoiding the problem of unscrupulous women having regular half-days off. After the first visit, a pregnant woman must be advised by a registered medical practitioner to go for antenatal care and will have an appointment card; she must not be 'unreasonably refused' time off to attend and must be paid as normal for that time. If her salary varies from week to week, she has to be paid the pro-rata rate of her average salary for the last 12 weeks. If an employer is dubious about a claim he can demand a certificate from a

GP, or from the hospital where the antenatal care is be given. If an employer does unreasonably refuse time off, to pay a pregnant employee properly, then an employee can take him to an industrial tribunal for a declaration of her rights for time off or the correct pay.

The Rights to Maternity Pay and to Return to Work Following Pregnancy

These two rights are linked. The preconditions for them are set down in S. 33 of the Act and are as follows:

(a) The employee must work up until the 11th week before the expected date of confinement.

(b) By the 11th week, she must have had at least 2 years' service with the employer.

(c) At least 21 days before she intends to cease work she must inform the employer that she intends to cease work and that she intends to return to work (if applicable). An employee should always say she will go back to work if she is in any doubt, as she can change her mind later if she wants to, whereas she cannot change her mind the other way. This notification of her intention to cease work can be oral or in writing, but the undertaking to return to work must be in writing. If requested, the employee must provide a certificate from her GP stating the expected week of confinement. An employee cannot stop work before the 11th week, but she can stop later and she would still, then, have the right to 6 weeks' maternity pay which, as defined in S. 35 is nine-tenths normal wages less any maternity allowance payable, and this applies whether or not the employee claims the maternity allowance (an employee would be very foolish not to do so!). If an

(b) Having entered into employment:

(i) in affording access to opportunities for promotion, transfer or training or any other benefits, facilities or services;

(ii) in dismissing or subjecting the person to any other detriment, e.g. transfer.

If anyone feels unfairly treated on grounds of sexual or racial discrimination, they are entitled to go to an industrial tribunal which can make a compensatory award against the employer concerned. Thus very great care is needed in formulating job advertisements, in conducting shortlisting and interviewing for jobs, and in the treatment and promotion of staff in order to ensure that no conscious or unconscious, tangible or implied discrimination takes place. Clear, brief notes should be made on all job applications as to why a candidate was not shortlisted or why she did not get the job at an interview, in order to provide protection against claims from aggrieved applicants. The Codes of Practice issued by the Equal Opportunities Commission and the Commission for Racial Equality should be read carefully by all health care managers.

Miscellaneous Employment Protection Rights

There are a number of other rights which employees legally have and of which health care managers need to be aware:

1. All employees should be given a statutory statement of their employment particulars before they have been employed for over 13 weeks and they should be notified of any changes after a further 4 weeks.
2. Employees have the right to receive an itemized pay statement showing gross pay, all deductions and the net pay figure. If gross pay is compiled

from different tasks—overtime, on-call, etc.—then these should be shown separately as well as in the total. If any unnotified deductions are made, then an industrial tribunal can award up to 13 weeks of unnotified deductions as a penalty (S. 8 EPCA).

3. If there is no work for the employees then those with more than 4 weeks' employment are entitled to receive a maximum of £10.50 per day from the State on a maximum of 5 days in any period of 3 months (S. 12 EPCA). This does not apply where the workless day has been caused by industrial action.
4. Employees are protected from having action short of dismissal taken against them on the grounds of trade union membership. There is no minimum length of service for this protection and theoretically no maximum limit on the compensation that can be awarded (S. 23 EPCA). This would apply to such issues as giving trade union members smaller pay increases, not promoting them, or transferring them to less favourable work.
5. Employees have the right not to be compelled to become a member of a trade union unless there is a closed shop agreement in existence for which there needs to have been an 80% vote in favour, this percentage being of all those eligible to vote and not just those who do vote.
6. Officials of recognized independent trade unions are entitled to reasonable time off with pay to carry out official duties concerned with employer/employee matters and for training (S. 27 EPCA).
7. Trade union members have the right to unpaid time off to carry on trade union activities, such as

attending conferences as a delegate, but they are not allowed time off to attend local union meetings unless this has been locally negotiated for employees (S. 28 EPCA).

8. Employees who carry out public duties are entitled to unpaid time off, e.g. for being a JP, a local health or water authority member, attending tribunals, or being a school or college governor.
9. Under the Truck Acts manual employees are entitled to be paid weekly in cash.
10. Minimum notice rights. After 4 weeks' service, an employee is entitled to 1 week's notice. After 2 years he is entitled to 2 weeks' notice and thereafter an additional week's notice for each complete year of service up to a maximum of 12 weeks after 12 years' continuous service.
11. After 26 weeks' service, an employee is entitled to written reasons for dismissal. If inaccurate, untrue, or inadequate reasons are given for a dismissal, an employee can be awarded 2 weeks' pay by an industrial tribunal with no maximum limit on the amount of a week's pay.
12. Transfer of Undertaking (Protection of Employment) Regulations. These only apply to the transfer of a business as a going concern, not to the sale of shares. Where a new owner steps into an old owner's shoes and inherits, *inter alia,* all the employment contracts existing immediately before the time of the transfer, and the collective agreements are also transferred, then the new employer is obliged to consult the unions about the effects of a change of ownership.
13. Where a business becomes insolvent an employee's rights to back pay or redundancy payments are

protected by payments from the central government redundancy fund.

14. Right to Statutory Sick Pay (SSP). The Social Security and Housing Benefits Act, 1982 places an obligation on employers to pay a fixed rate during the initial period of an employee's illness which is then reclaimed from the government. At present SSP is paid for up to 8 weeks in any one tax year and the rates paid are based on a sliding scale of normal earnings.

Individual Action

Going on strike is the most serious breach of contract that an employee can commit and it renders him liable to summary dismissal (S. 62 EPCA). The only situations in which an employee could claim unfair dismissal at an industrial tribunal, after being dismissed for taking strike action, would be:

1. If any other employee who was also on strike on that day was not dismissed.
2. If any other employee who was also on strike on that day, and was dismissed, had been offered re-engagement, and the complainant had not, within 3 months of the date of dismissal.

Trade Union Action

A trade union is a quasi-legal entity which can be sued in certain circumstances, but not in all. It is almost impossible for a trade union engaged in industrial action not to breach some part of the common law. Most notably, it may be guilty of intimidation, conspiracy, or procuring a breach of contract, all of which are common law torts. However, acts done in contemplation or futherance of a trade dispute are granted immunity from actions of tort by S. 13 of the 1974 Trade Union and Labour Relations Act if they induce members to break or interfere with a contract or threaten to do so, as long as:

1. It has held a ballot to make the action official under S. 10 of the 1984 Trade Union Act. The ballot must be conducted in secret and on paper and a 51% majority is required of those who vote. The question asked on the ballot paper must be capable of being answered by yes or no. If the ballot does not fulfil all these criteria the union loses its legal indemnity from being sued for damages by an employer.
2. It is not secondary action outside the terms of S. 17 (3), (4) and (5) of the 1980 Employment Act. This only allows secondary action which interferes with contracts between the employer involved in the trade dispute and his first supplier and first customers, but it may be extended to an associated employer if that employer is performing the contract for the employer who is in dispute.

The amount of damages recoverable is limited by the number of members in a trade union but there is a limit of £50 000 on any one occasion for unions with over 100 000 members. If the union refuses to pay, its funds can be sequestrated and removed from the control of the union officials to the control of a court-appointed sequestrator, as happened in the 1984/5 Miners' Strike.

Control Law

All managers in health care should have a basic understanding of contract law, since they are likely to be involved in taking decisions about which company supplies the forms, chemicals, reagents, drugs and X-ray film which are used and the choice of the machines and equipment that utilize these supplies.

Various things are necessary before a contract exists. There needs to be (1) an offer of goods or services, (2) an acceptance of that offer, (3) consideration, (4) an intention on the part of both parties to be legally bound and create legal relations, and (5) contractual capacity.

1. An offer is a promise to be bound to do something, or provide something, provided specified terms are accepted. An offer does not have to be made on a one-to-one basis—as was determined in the 1893 case of Carlill v. Carbolic Smoke Ball Co. The company had advertised that if anybody caught influenza after using their product they would pay them £100. Mrs Carlill claimed and it was held that she was not entitled to the money. Such advertisements are often held to be mere 'puffs', too widely aimed to be intended to create legal relations, but as the company had deposited £1000 with a bank to show its sincerity it was held to be liable. An invitation to treat is not an offer. Items displayed with a price tag in a shop window do not comprise an offer, the price tag is an invitation for anyone to make an offer to buy at that price. The 1952 case of the Pharmaceutical Society v. Boots the Chemist was brought because Boots sold controlled drugs in their first supermarket style shops and at the time these could only be sold by a qualified pharmacist. As a result, Boots put qualified pharmacists on their payment tills and this was held to be legal as the offer was deemed to be made at the till, when customers offered to buy the drugs at the price advertised.

2. Acceptance of an offer may be expressed or inferred. An expressed acceptance would be saying 'yes' to an offer. An inferred acceptance would be if you went away and returned with a cheque for the amount for which the object of service was offered. You cannot accept an offer by saying nothing or doing nothing, but an oral acceptance is sufficient, such as the ordering of goods by telephone. However, you

must accept an offer in the manner which is no less efficient than that specified, e.g. if an advert says an acceptance must be in writing then it must be in writing. The communication of your acceptance of an offer is valid when it is received, except when posted, regardless of whether it arrives, unless the offer specifies that the acceptance must be *received* in writing. Unless an acceptance is sent by recorded delivery it would obviously be hard to prove postage.

3. Any offer stays alive until it is revoked. This can be done either by making a counter-offer, for example, at a higher or lower price; by the lapse of time, for instance, the offer being limited to 14 days; by deliberately revoking an offer at any time before its acceptance; or by revoking an acceptance before it becomes valid, for example by sending a telex between posting and arrival. It is necessary to have knowledge of an offer before it can be accepted, for example you could not claim a discount on new equipment after ordering it because you were unaware at the time of ordering it that a discount was being offered.

4. Consideration. This is what one person gives in return for what is being given, and is usually money, but does not have to be, e.g. a bartering system. The consideration given must be for an adequate amount.

5. In order to create a legally binding contract, there must be an intention to create legal relations and the parties must have the capacity to contract. Anyone over 18 can enter into a contract but minors under 18 must have the consent of a parent or guardian except in exceptional circumstances. People suffering from mental incapacity or insanity are also excluded from entering contracts under the terms of the Mental Health Act. Companies are legal entities and have contractual capacity, but they are limited to entering contracts only for the purposes for which the

company was set up. These are laid down in the Object Clause of a company's Articles of Association which states the purposes for which the company has been created and limits its contractual capacity to very definite areas. If a company exceeds its Object Clause it is said to be *ultra vires* or to have exceeded its powers. The Company can be sued for doing this, but it cannot itself sue someone else for not supplying goods or services if it has done this.

6. Contracts. The terms of a contract can be purely oral and word of mouth is just as good, in theory, as being in writing, but it is obviously much safer to have a written contract. Certain contracts have, by law, to be in writing (land dispositions, trusts), and some must be evidenced in writing as we have seen earlier, in that everyone must be given a written contract of employment by the end of their 13th week in employment. The terms of a contract can be expressed or implied, and there are three ways to imply:

(a) *By custom.* For example, if a contract is silent as to the way the goods are to be delivered, then one would look at the trade custom and that would define how they should be delivered.

(b) *By statute.* In the absence of terms to the contrary in the contract, then the relevant statute law automatically applies, e.g. S. 49 of the 1978 EPCA defining minimum periods of notice, or S. 14 of the 1979 Sale of Goods Act which lays down that goods being sold will be fit for their purpose and of merchantable quality, including second-hand goods.

(c) *By courts.* Judgements often precede statutes being drawn up by governments, e.g. Lister v. Romford Ice Co. (1957), where it was held that an employee who ran his father over whilst driving a company lorry had an implied duty of good faith and fidelity and should have shown reasonable skill and care.

Vitiating Elements

These elements are ones that can make a contract invalid and ineffectual.

Mistake

There are three types of mistakes, common, mutual and unilateral, and they mean that a contract is entered into by mistake as to the subject-matter of the contract, or to carry out something which is not capable of being carried out.

Misrepresentation

There are two types:

1. Deliberate misrepresentation: where duress or threats were used, say by a large organisation on a small one, to get the small organisation to enter into a contract against its will.
2. Innocent misrepresentation: where a statement, made about the facts on which the contract is being drawn up, induces a party to enter into the contract and is later found to be incorrect. Misrepresentation is not normally possible by silence except in three situations:
    (a) By being silent about changes to earlier positive representations, e.g. 'this machine is fully guaranteed for five years', but the guarantee is reduced during negotiations to one year and the salesman does not tell the buyer. Any changes to the subject matter of a contract must be constantly updated during negotiations.

(b) Contracts of an *uberrimae fidei* ('of the utmost good faith') nature, such as insurance contracts, where one party, the proposer, knows more than the other and, therefore, full and frank disclosure of all facts material to a contract must be made by a proposer.

(c) Fiduciary relationships, where trusts or trustees are involved; who are bound by other rules apart from the contract.

Misrepresentations must induce one party into a contract into which they would not otherwise have entered and, again, there are three types:

1. Fraudulent: where you know or are reckless to the fact that the statement was incorrect.
2. Negligent: where you ought to have known that the statement was incorrect.
3. Innocent: where you could not possibly have known the statement was incorrect.

The remedies for misrepresentation are that a fraudulent statement rescinds the contract and restores the parties' prior status—*restitutio in integrum*. However, under the terms of the 1967 Misrepresentations Act, damages can be awarded in lieu of rescission and damages are also awarded for negligent or innocent misrepresentation.

Void Contracts

Any restraint of trade clauses are *prima facie* void, unless they are reasonable to the interests of the parties concerned and the general public. There are three fundamental conditions which have to be followed before restrictive covenants are allowed in employment contracts:

(a) They must be reasonable for the protection of the employer's business interests, e.g. customer goodwill, trade secrets.

(b) They must not be unnecessarily wide with regard to geographical area or time.

(c) An employee cannot be prevented from exercising his skill and experience.

Great care is, therefore, necessary from both health care managers and their suppliers in ensuring that legally binding contracts are properly drawn up and entered into.

Data Protection Act 1984

The other major area of legislation which health care managers need to be aware of is the Data Protection Act, which became law on 12 July, 1984.

The Act is designed to enable the UK to ratify the Council of Europe's 1983 convention for the protection of individuals, with regard to automatic processing of personal data, and to embrace CECD guidelines on the protection of privacy and trans-border flows of personal data. The Act is based upon the data protection principles established by the Council of Europe and, without this Act, there was a danger of other countries restricting the flow of personal data to the UK. This Act also meets the concern that arises from the threat which misuse of the power of computing equipment might pose to individuals; this derives from the ability of computing systems to store vast amounts of data, to manipulate data at high speeds and, with associated communications systems, to give access to data from locations far from the site where the data are stored.

Purpose of the Act

The Act covers personal data (i.e. data which can be identified as relating to a living individual) held in a form that can be processed automatically (i.e. by equipment in response to instructions given for the purpose). Such personal data and their uses will need to be registered with a Data

Protection Registrar, presently E.J. Howe, and will need to be open to access by the individual on request. The Act sets out to achieve the following:

(a) To give data subjects, people whose names and identities are held on a computer file, certain legal rights, such as access to data of which they are the subject and compensation where damage has resulted due to the personal data held;

(b) To establish a Data Protection Registrar whose functions will include:

— maintaining a register of all personal data users and computer bureaux, unless they are specifically exempted;

— [hang-1where necessary, using his statutory powers to enforce compliance with the Act;

— [hang-1considering any complaint that any of the data protection principles of any provision of the Act are being contravened.

(c) To set up a tribunal to consider appeals by data users in dispute with the Registrar.

Main Features

The Act is not intended to prevent the holding and use of personal data, but to ensure that certain standards are maintained.

The data user (i.e. the person who controls the contents and use of personal data), is responsible for the registration and proper use of the files according to eight principles laid down in the Act. All eight principles apply to a data user. A bureau, which processes data on behalf of a user, is governed only by the eighth principle.

(a) The information to be contained in personal data

shall be obtained, and personal data shall be processed, fairly and lawfully.

(b) Personal data shall be held only for one or more specified and lawful purposes.

(c) Personal data held for any purpose shall not be used or disclosed in any manner incompatible with that purpose (i.e. used or disclosed only in accordance with the data user's register entry).

(d) Personal data held for any purpose shall be adequate, relevant and not excessive in relation with that purpose.

(e) Personal data shall be accurate and, where necessary, kept up-to-date.

(f) Personal data held for any purpose shall not be kept for longer than is necessary for the purpose.

(g) An individual shall be entitled:

  (i) At reasonable intervals and without undue delay or expense, to be informed by any data user whether he holds personal data of which that individual is the subject, and to have access to any such data held by a data user.

  (ii) Where appropriate to have such data corrected or erased.

(h) Appropriate security measures shall be taken against unauthorized access to, or alteration, disclosure or destruction of, personal data, and against accidental loss or destruction of personal data. Failure to comply with the Act can lead to criminal or civil proceedings or both.

Key Definitions

The Act is concerned with personal data held on data subjects by data users and computer bureaux.

(a) *Personal data* is data consisting of information which relates to a living individual who can be identified from the information, including any expression of opinion about the individual but not any indication of the intentions of the data user in respect of that individual.

— 'Information which relates to': whether an item of information 'relates to' an individual is a question of fact which must be determined in the particular.

— 'A living individual': if the subject is dead or is not a subject (e.g. if it is a company) the information cannot constitute personal data.

— 'Can be identified': the identification may be direct (e.g. where the subject's name is recorded as part of the data) or indirect (e.g. where the data contain a code from which, by reference to a separate list in your possession, the subject can be identified).

— 'Not any indication of the intentions': it is only your intentions which are excluded, not those of third parties.

(b) *Data subjects* are individuals who are subjects of personal data.

— 'An individual': a data subject need not be a United Kingdom resident. A company is not an individual and cannot be a data subject. However, persons in business on their own account (sole traders) are individuals and therefore can be data subjects.

(c) *Data users* are persons who hold data for automatic processing and control the contents and use of the data. A person *holds data* if:

— The data form part of a collection of data processed or intended to be processed by or on behalf of that person (individual as denned above).

— That person (either alone or jointly or in common with other persons) controls the content and use of the data comprised in the collection.

— The data are in a form in which they have been or are intended to be processed or in a form into which they have been converted after being so processed and with a view to being processed on a subsequent occasion.

— 'By and on behalf of: to be a data user you need not own a computer or do any processing yourself. If data are processed on your behalf (e.g. by a computer bureau) you may be a data user.

— 'Jointly or in common': covers the situation where control is exercised by a number of persons acting together or by each of a group of persons.

— 'Controls': this is a vital element in the definition. You are not a data user and do not 'hold' data unless you are entitled to take the final decision as to the information which is to be recorded and as to the purposes for which the data are to be used.

— The data are in the form etc.': data which has been processed and then converted into a different form remains regulated by the Act if there is a prospect of processing the data automatically again in the future.

Note. The data user is the person or organisation which *controls* the data content and use. Anyone who has an arrangement, no matter how informal, to let a third party use his/her machine as a back-up during system failure must register as a user and bureau.

(d) *A computer bureau* exists where a person, as agent for others, causes data to be processed or allows other persons to use equipment in his possession for processing.

(e) *Processing,* in relation to data, means amending, augmenting, deleting or rearranging the data or extracting the information constituting the data and in the case of personal data, means performing any of these operations by reference to the data subject. This should not be construed as applying to any operation performed only for the purpose of preparing the text of documents.

— 'processing': no upper or lower limit of size or number of records is given and thus all systems which contain personal data must be registered.

— 'extracting the information': operations such as transmission, display and printing are covered since, in each case, extraction is an element of the operation.

Note. The exclusion of text preparation does not exclude word processing *per se.* Each system must be assessed to determine whether registration is required.

(f) *Disclosing,* in relation to data, includes disclosing information extracted from the data and where the identification of the individual who is the subject of personal data depends partly on the information in possession of the data user.

Note. The medium of disclosure is not limited—it could be oral or handwritten as well as printed or displayed on a screen. There is, however, no disclosure if the identification of the subject of the personal details is dependent on other information in the possession of the data user which is not itself disclosed.

(g) The term 'computer' is not defined in the Act but the definition of data refers to processing 'by equipment operating automatically in response to instructions given for that purpose.'

Impact on Data Users

The Act is based on eight data protection principles as set out in Schedule 1 to the Act. The Act affects users of personal data as follows:

(a) *Registration* is required of *all* applications which process personal data automatically, unless specifically exempted.

(b) *Personal data collected* must have been obtained:

— fairly and lawfully (principle 1);

— from a source described in the registered entry.

(c) *Personal data held* must be:

— described in the registered entry;

— held for one or more lawful purposes specified in the registered entry (principle 2);

— adequate, relevant and not excessive for the purpose for which they are held (principle 4);

— accurate and, where necessary, kept up-to-date (principle 5);

— kept no longer than is necessary for the purpose for which they are maintained (principle 6);

— secure against unauthorized access, alteration, disclosure or destruction, and against accidental loss or destruction (principle 8).

(d) *Dissemination of personal data* must only be:

- for the purpose described in the registered entry (principle 3);
- allowed by a computer bureau with the prior authority of the person for whom the bureau services are being provided;
- to a country or territory outside the UK if named in the registered entry.

(e) *Personal data subject's rights* include:

- entitlement to know, within 40 days of a request, whether the data user holds data of which the individual is the subject (principle 7);
- the right within 40 days of a request, to a copy of such data in an intelligible form;
- entitlement to apply to have personal data corrected or erased, where appropriate (principle 7);
- compensation where the subject has suffered damage through the inaccuracy, loss or unauthorized disclosure of personal data.

Registration

Unless exempted from registration, any person who holds personal data for automatic processing must have an appropriate entry in the register of data users. The following particulars are required:

(a) Name and address of data user.

(b) A description of the personal data held and the purpose for which the data are to held or used.

(c) A description of the source(s) from which the data might be obtained.

(d) The person(s) to whom the data might be disclosed.

(e) The name of any country or territory outside the UK to which the data might be transferred directly or indirectly.

(f) One or more addresses for the receipt of requests from data subjects for access to the data.

During March, 1985, the Data Protection Registrar conducted pilot trials on his proposed Data Registration Form. The Wessex Regional Health Authority was involved in these and a number of points of concern arose:

— the form was considerably larger and more complex than expected;

— the time taken to complete the forms is substantial;

— the standard entries which have been proposed by the Registrar do not cover a large percentage of the data items and purposes of NHS clinical, investigative and surveillance systems.

Exemptions

The degree of exemption given by the Act varies and covers a number of categories. The exemptions most relevant are outlined below:

(a) Exemption from registration, non-disclosure provisions, subject access provisions, and provisions relating to compensation, rectification and erasure.

(i) Payroll and accounts personal data qualify where they are held only for the payment of remuneration, pensions etc. or for keeping accounts for ensuring that the requisite payments are made by or to the data user. Use of personal data for making financial or management forecasts is also permitted,

(ii) Distribution of articles—personal data used for this purpose are exempt provided:

— the data consist only of the data subjects' names, addresses or other particulars necessary for effecting the distribution, and the data subject has been asked and agrees to these data being held.

(iii) Other Acts of parliament—these may require personal data to be disclosed.

(b) Exemption from the subject access provisions:

(i) Regulation of financial services.

(ii) Statistical preparation and research—provided that the results are not made available in a form that identifies the data subject.

(iii) Consumer Credit Act 1974.

(iv) Legal professional privilege.

(v) Back-up copies of personal data that are kept solely for replacing other data in the event of their loss are exempt,

(vi) Offences under other Acts of parliament.

(c) Exemption from the non-disclosure provision:

(i) Disclosure is permitted for obtaining legal advice or during legal proceedings or when required by any other enactments or court orders,

(ii) Where there is an urgent need to prevent injury or damage to health, disclosure of personal data is allowed,

(iii) In any case where data subjects have requested disclosure, the non-disclosure provisions will not apply.

Some Key Dates

12 September, 1984: a data subject may seek compensation through the Courts for any damage or associated distress suffered on or after this date.

September, 1985: registration commenced.

March, 1986: existing data users and computer bureaux must have applied for registration before this date. Holding of personal data by an unregistered person became a criminal offence. Registered data users became bound to operate within the terms of their registered entries. Data users became liable to pay compensation in respect of damage or associated distress suffered on or after this date by reason of inaccuracy of personal data.

September, 1987: The 'subject access' provisions come into force.

SUMMARY OF THE PROVISIONS OF THE HSW ACT, 1974

There are four main parts of the Act:

— health and safety in general
— medical aspects
— building regulations
— miscellaneous provisions.

Part 1

The objectives of the Act are to make work safer and healthier and to replace existing legislation with new regulations and codes of practice.

Section 2

This section makes it the duty of every employer to ensure, so far as is reasonably practicable, the health, safety and welfare at work of all employees. This is specifically related to plant, systems of work, use, handling, transport and storage of goods, place of work, safety training and supervision. In a sense, this adds criminal penalties to existing common law duties.

The section extends inspectors' powers to all types of circumstances except domestic services.

All employers of more than 5 employees must publish and abide by a written statement of safety policy. This must identify particular hazards and state the name of the manager with ultimate health and safety responsibility, and all others within the organisation with health and safety responsibilities. The statement must ensure that employees are made aware of hazards and what their own responsibilities are. It should refer to training needs and policy at all levels within the organisation.

Recognized trade unions may appoint safety representatives—this is important to the self-regulation and mutual responsibility philosophy of the Act. Employers must consult safety representatives with a view to making arrangements for joint co-operation in bringing about safe working conditions. If necessary, representatives can require the employer to set up Safety Committees. This is an extension of existing provisions under Mine Safety legislation which gave miners' representatives similar powers.

Section 3

This section places an obligation upon an employer to take reasonable care for the safety of persons who are not his employees, but who are likely to be affected by his operations, e.g. customers, patients, trespassers, sub-contractors, etc. For the first time the self-employed are given similar responsibilities.

Employers and self-employed must divulge information on health and safety matters to all persons affected by them.

Section 4

Under this section anyone in control of business premises must take reasonable care to see that the premises and any equipment are safe for people using them, whether or not they are employees.

Section 5

This section gives the person in control of business premises an obligation to use the best practicable means of preventing the emission of harmful or offensive substances into the air.

Section 6

Section 6 imposes a duty on the designers, manufacturers, importers and suppliers of any article or substance for use at work to ensure, so far as is reasonably practicable, that they are safely designed and adequately tested and all necessary information about their use is given.

It is made a statutory obligation for any person erecting or installing articles or equipment for use at work to do so safely.

Inspectors are given power to prosecute the manufacturers or designers of unsafe products. Again this adds criminal penalties to common law duties.

Section 7

This section places a responsibility upon employees to take reasonable care for their own and others' safety and to co-operate with their employers so far as is necessary to enable them to carry out their own safety obligations.

Section 8

The intentional or reckless interference with, or misuse of, safety devices or equipment required by law is made an offence.

Section 9

This section prohibits the employer from charging employees for safety devices and equipment which is required by law, e.g. masks, protective clothing, machine guards.

Sections 10-15

This part of the Act establishes the 'Health and Safety Commission' (HSC) and the 'Health and Safety Executive' (HSE) to oversee safety, health and welfare in all types and places of employment other than domestic service. Agricultural safety was later brought under the Commission's jurisdiction by the Employment Protection Act.

The Health and Safety Commission has 9 members. Three members are supplied by the unions, 3 by management, 2 represent local authorities and, since no-one can agree, one place remains unfilled. The chairman is appointed by the Secretary of State.

The Commission's duties include the provision of information and advice on health and safety and it can sponsor research and inquiries. It is a quasi-independent body, but is ultimately responsible to the Secretary of State for Employment.

The Secretary of State is empowered to make health and safety regulations.

Sections 16-17

The Health and Safety Commission is empowered to issue Codes of Safe Working Practice to explain how the general legal duties in the Act can be fulfilled. It is intended that these codes of practice should give an indication of basic statutory requirements, but non-compliance with a code of practice is not in itself an offence. Under Section 17 an employer can escape liability by showing that he has done his best to fulfil his duties in some other appropriate fashion.

Sections 18-28

This part of the Act concerns enforcement and the powers and duties of inspectors. The enforcement of the Act is made the responsibility of the Executive, although the Secretary of State may require other bodies, in particular local authorities, to undertake particular aspects of the work.

Inspectors have a right of entry to conduct enquiries and investigations on the premises. An inspector may direct that equipment or premises are left undisturbed and may take samples. He can require information to be given by particular individuals.

Under Section 21 he may serve a time-limited Improvement Notice to remedy any breach of the Act, while under Section 22 an inspector may serve a Prohibition Notice if there is an imminent risk of serious personal injury. This notice orders the particular activity to stop until the notice has been complied with. Section 23 states that a notice may give a specific remedy, it may require compliance with a code of practice or give the person responsible the choice of remedial actions. Alternatively, the recipient of the notice may be left to decide himself how the breach should be remedied. Appeals against notices are made to an industrial tribunal.

Inspectors are given the power under Section 25 to seize and make harmless any articles or substances they believe to be dangerous, but they must give a full report to the person responsible for them. Inspectors are indemnified by the Act for any liability they may incur. Section 28 is again evidence of the underlying philosophy of the Act towards mutual responsibility in that it requires the inspector to give factual information he may have obtained about safety risks and his action, to the employees or their representatives, as well as the employer.

Prosecutions under the Act are heard in the Magistrates' Court or, in more serious cases, the Crown Court.

Sections 29-32

This part of the Act made special provision for agriculture. As stated above, agricultural health and safety did not originally come under the Health and Safety Commission. This has now been remedied by the Employment Protection Act.

Sections 33-42

This part of the Act specifies the nature of criminal proceedings under the Act. The penalties for breaches of the statutory requirements within the Act are very realistic—a fine of up to £1000 for breaches of administrative requirements and unlimited fines for refusal to comply with improvement or prohibition notices. Daily penalties for continued non-compliance may also be made. The penalty of imprisonment is imposed for the first time and it is likely to be used in cases of recklessness and severe neglect. An interesting reversal of general common law principles is that Section 40 places upon the person charged the burden of proof that all practicable steps have been taken to fulfil the Act's requirements.

The Reminder of the Act

The Crown is exempt from the enforcement provisions

of the Act. However, this 'Crown Immunity' has been removed from NHS authorities by the NHS (Amendment) Act, 1986 and applies to health authorities for the first time (Sections 21-25 and 33-42 of the 1974 Act).

In Part II of the Act the Employment Medical Advisory Service is brought under the Health and Safety Commission.

Part III concerns the Building Regulations and the Amendment of Building (Scotland) Act, 1959, widens the scope of existing legislation and changes administrative arrangements. Crown buildings are brought under statutory control.

Part IV of the Act covers the co-ordination of the activities of the HSE and the National Radiological Protection Board. Responsibility for fire precautions and means of escape are transferred to fire authorities.

The general obligations of the Act, which place duties on all employers (with the exception of those of domestic servants) came into force at the beginning of April 1975. The general umbrella of the Act provides for an interaction of responsibility for the individuals and organisations associated with work, or touched by its immediate consequences. Thus the employer has a duty to his employees with regard to their health and safety and those employees have a duty to one another. The general public are also entitled to a duty of care in terms of safety and health by people carrying out work activities. This includes patients, visitors of all kinds and on-site contractors. A person carrying on an inherently dangerous activity or one that is a threat to health if something goes wrong is obliged to inform not only his workers but also all relevant third parties including the local population if necessary. In many organisations this is achieved by the use of warning notices which frequently prohibit entry to premises by unauthorized personnel.

There is a requirement for importers, manufacturers, designers and suppliers of any machinery, plant or substance, to ensure it is in a safe condition when properly used, before it arrives at the premises and is brought into use.

In fulfilling all such duties prescribed by the Act the test is that of what is 'reasonably practicable' to achieve. It could be argued that these general duties merely enact the employer's common law obligations. The test of 'reasonably practicable' places the responsibility for health and safety squarely on the individual employer and/or employee rather than on adherence to an externally imposed regulation. In fulfilling both the letter and the spirit of the law the employer would be wise to consider all available information and experience, having regard to normal industrial practice and the particular safety considerations of all his work practices. He may consult experts for advice such as the HSE, the British Safety Council, or any other body with expertise and he is obliged to consult the representatives of his workforce if so requested.

Lewis argues that the words 'reasonably practicable' do not mean that the employer must do everything that is physically possible to safeguard employees, only that the risks be weighed against the trouble and expense of eliminating or reducing them. This introduces the notion of economic evaluation into local safety policy and code-making and is a consideration to which we will return later in this study.

Safety Policies

It is in the nature of enabling legislation that powers are given to the Secretary of State for the Environment to introduce statutory Codes of Practice, to meet health and safety at work contingencies as they arise, and to amend or repeal outdated ones. Clearly this is not an adequate means of controlling all safety practice at organisational levels and, as we have seen, responsibility is given to the employer by introducing the concept of self-regulation into health and safety management.

The basis of this is the written safety policy which the Employer has to compile due to the specific duty laid on him by Section 2 (3) of the Act. This calls for every employer to prepare and, as often as may be appropriate, revise, a written statement of his general policy with respect to the health and safety at work of his employees and the organisation and arrangements for the time being in force for carrying out that policy. He has a duty to bring the statement and any revision of it to the notice of all his employees.

'A safety policy is an essential part of self-regulation', said the Health Services Advisory Committee (HSAC). 'It should be more than writing on a piece of paper. It gives an opportunity to demonstrate that the employer accepts that a commitment to health and safety is an integral part of the organisation of an undertaking and that management at the highest level means to ensure that this commitment will be translated into effective action. It is important that the policy reflects the uniqueness and the special needs of the organisation for whom it is written. The document cannot be bought or borrowed nor can it be written by outside consultants or inspectors.'

The complexities of the NHS require that several health and safety policies be written appropriate to the various levels and specialism within the service. The HSAC recommends a three-part safety policy to include the overall policy of the authority, the policy of each officer in charge of a specialism and the policy related to each geographical unit.

In each case the policy should be clear and specific as to its meaning and to the means whereby safe practices are to be maintained. For example, it should identify not only the safety training to be given to staff but should state the name or post of the designated trainer. The policy should specify the means of its own review, again identifying the responsible person. Other matters dealt with will include joint consultation and liaison arrangements between staff groups and the employers, and/or other affected parties, such as adjacent employers with whom liaison is required, such as medical schools.

The policy will show the chosen organisation within the district from the authority downwards. It would seem sensible to identify the district general manager (DGM) as overall co-ordinator for the policy within the district, and for such further regulations as may from time to time be issued by the Health and Safety Commission and Executive and the DHSS. The unit general managers might be expected to act on behalf of the DGM at unit level and for this purpose might be designated safety co-ordinators.

The need for co-ordination is illustrated particularly by the examples of codes and rules which apply across a number of Departments:

- the prevention of cross-infection
- radiological protection rules
- Code of Protection on the Prevention of Infection in Clinical Laboratories and Post-Mortem Rooms—the Howie Report
- fire prevention policy
- clinical waste policy
- medical gases

- DHSS health technical memoranda
- health building notes and design guides
- health and safety policy for contractors
- hazard notices, safety information bulletins, health equipment information.

Heads of department, as managers, are responsible for the health and safety of the staff they supervise and the workplaces they control. The head of department will normally be the safety supervisor but this function can be delegated to a senior subordinate. Safety supervisors are responsible for preparing a departmental safety policy which should be agreed with the safety co-ordinator before being issued to all staff in the department. Even where the duty of safety supervisor is delegated it will not remove the ultimate responsibility for health and safety which is placed upon heads of department and line managers. A safety supervisor who is a subordinate should keep his head of department fully informed on representations made by the trade unions and should only act with his knowledge and consent. The names of safety supervisors should be displayed on departmental notice boards.

Following these general issues come the codes of practice that relate to hazardous or potentially hazardous work. An example of such a hazard arises when nursing and/or investigating a patient with an infectious disease. The protocol of a barrier nursing method constitutes such a code. As an HSW Act code of practice, however, it should state the name of the person responsible for supervising the training and compliance with the code, usually the immediate supervisor, and give the names or agencies from whom help and advice can be obtained.

The HSAC give the following headings, in a checklist, for identifying matters to be covered in the safety policy:

1. The policy statement—management intention.
2. The organisation for health and safety—how it will be carried out.
3. Arrangements for health and safety.

These would cover specific topics such as:

- Training—who needs it and who does it
- Safe systems of work
- Environmental control
- Safe place of work
- Machinery and plant
- Noise and vibration
- Radiation
- Dust
- Toxic materials
- Gases
- Infection risks
- Waste disposal
- Transport
- Violence
- Internal communication
- Fire
- Medical facilities and welfare
- Records
- Emergency procedures
- Monitoring at the work place

Having established a policy, monitoring of its effectiveness is essential. Codes of practice may be unworkable or become so due to technological or organisational change and thus their regular supervision and updating is an essential task for the safety supervisor. A failure to observe any provision of an approved code of practice is not in itself a criminal offence. However, such codes are admissible in evidence and proof of failure to comply with a code will demonstrate that all reasonably practicable measures had not been taken, unless it could be proved that the code itself was unworkable.

Criminal proceedings may arise in two circumstances. Where an employer fails to respond adequately to an improvement or prohibition notice or where there is an accident or other dangerous occurrence which is reported to the HSE. In the latter case a criminal action by the HSE may be followed by civil action by injured parties to recover damages from those deemed to have been responsible. Since, under the Civil Evidence Act, 1968, a conviction for a criminal offence is admissible in civil proceedings as evidence that the person so convicted committed the offence, the civil action will invariably await the outcome of any criminal prosecution. Penalties under the Act may be a fine up to £1000 for most offences in summary proceedings (before magistrates) and up to two years' imprisonment coupled with an unlimited fine if there is a prosecution or indictment in a higher court.

Role of the Safety Supervisor

Within our model of health and safety we see that detailed responsibilities within individual departments are vested with safety supervisors who are usually the heads of those departments. Their main responsibilities are:

1. To identify potential hazards in their own area and

to bring them to the attention of the safety co-ordinator (UGM) if they are unable to remedy the problem.

2. To receive representations in the first instance from safety representatives.
3. To liaise with specialist staff whose work relates to health and safety in relation to their own area.
4. To advise the safety co-ordinator (UGM) on matters arising from accident reports and to comment on representations made by the safety representatives. Strictly it is for heads of departments to report incidents under the Injuries, Diseases and Dangerous Occurences Regulations, 1986 (RIDDOR)
5. To assist the safety co-ordinator in discussions with the Health and Safety Executive's inspectors.
6. To organise and carry out safety audits.
7. To assist in implementing any required changes including, where appropriate, drawing up approved work procedures and ensuring that staff know and understand them.

Safety Representatives

Under the HSW Act Section 2 (4-7) an independent trade union recognized by an employer may appoint safety representatives to represent all or part of the workforce employed by the employer concerned. One of the functions of this statutory safety representative is that of carrying out safety inspections to check the effectiveness of health and safety measures in his workplace. All employers, under the Act, have a legal duty to consult safety representatives on the arrangements made for the maintenance and improvement of health and safety. The aim is for the employer to introduce and maintain systems and procedures which will enable him to co-operate effectively with his employees in matters affecting their health and safety at work.

A safety representative may carry out:

1. A general inspection (at not more than 3-monthly intervals).
2. An inspection following a change in conditions of work, or where new information is published on a hazard relevant to the workplace.
3. An inspection consequent to a notifiable accident, occurrence or disease.
4. The inspection of statutory documents relating to health, safety and welfare.

Within the NHS, employing authorities should accord safety representatives, appointed by bodies represented on the staff side of the Whitley Council (or other nationally recognized negotiating bodies) the rights and facilities described in the Regulations. Similar rights and facilities should also be granted to appointees of any other staff organisation that satisfies the definition of a 'recognized trade union'. That is to say recognized by an employer for the purpose of collective bargaining and independent of the domination and control of an employer. Appointments of safety representatives by such unions must be notified to management in writing. They will be granted time off with pay to perform their functions and to undergo appropriate training. The number of representatives appointed should be the number needed to carry out their function effectively. Problems can arise when more than one trade union is involved in a single department. Such difficulties may be resolved through normal local negotiating machinery. There is no legal right to appoint safety representatives in departments or units where no recognized trade union exists.

However, the lack of safety representatives in no way reduces management's responsibilities. Indeed, even greater vigilance will be called for in such circumstances. Safety representatives should be seen as allies not enemies by a manager and a fruitful co-operative relationship should be developed with them which should benefit all staff in the department.

Safety representatives will not be liable to civil or criminal proceedings so long as they have been correctly appointed in writing, are carrying out the functions allocated to them under the Regulations and are making appropriate provision in consequence of these functions. Nothing in the Regulations will diminish the employer's obligation under the Act.

Functions of Safety Representatives

The functions of the safety representatives will include:

1. Representing staff in consultation with management under Section 2 (6) of the Act.
2. Representing his members on any general or specific matter affecting their health and safety.
3. Representing those people employed at his place of work on general matters affecting their health and safety.
4. Carrying out inspections.
5. Representing his members in consultation with officers of the Health and Safety Executive and any other enforcing authority.
6. Receiving information from Inspectors (Section 28 (8) of the Act).
7. Attending meetings of the Safety Committee, when required.

It should be noted that these functions do not impose a duty on safety representatives.

Safety Officer

The term 'safety officer' does not appear in the literature except as a generic term which might equally apply to any of the above safety roles, namely safety co-ordinator, safety supervisor or safety representative. It could equally apply to a safety adviser who has the quite different role of that of an expert who may be retained to advise either side on safety matters. We therefore recommend that the term 'safety officer' is deleted since its use is often misleading.

Safety Committees

Under Section 9(1) and (2) of the Regulations which interpret Section 2 (7) of the HSW Act 1974, if any two safety representatives request, in writing, that a safety committee be set up, the employer, after consultation with those representatives and the representatives of other appropriate trade unions, shall establish the committee within 3 months. The composition of the committee shall be displayed in a notice at the workplace. The Commission favours discussion and negotiation between employers and safety representatives to establish the most effective way of interpreting this section of the Act. They believe that safety committees are more likely to prove effective where their work is related to a single establishment (i.e. unit) rather than a collection of geographically distinct places (i.e. district), although the usefulness of the 'district' committee is not entirely discounted.

Objectives and Functions of Safety Committees

Safety committees have the function of keeping under review the measures taken to ensure the health and safety at work of the employees. An objective should be the promotion of co-operation between employers and employees in instigating, developing and carrying out measures to ensure the health and safety at work of the employees. The committee would also act in an advisory capacity to management, in particular, with regard to the operation of the authority's health and safety policy.

Particular functions for, say, a District Health and Safety Committee might be to:

- review accident and ill health records
- consider reports on incidents, dangerous occurrences and near misses
- ensure standards of compliance with legal requirements, Crown Improvement and Prohibition Notices
- monitor progress on drawing up codes of practice
- review the extent to which long term objectives have been met within agreed time scales
- identify those areas in need of improvement
- receive regular reports from the Unit Safety Committees
- maintain all statutory records.

Other functions for safety committees as recommended by the HSC include:

- examination of safety audit reports
- consideration of Inspectors' reports
- consideration of reports from Safety Representatives
- assistance in the development of works safety rules and safe systems of work
- a watch on the effectiveness of the safety content of employee training
- a watch on the adequacy of safety and health communication and publicity in the workplace

— the provision of a link with the appropriate inspectorates of the enforcing authority.Membership of the Safety Committee

The membership of a safety committee should reflect the tasks it has to perform. We can find nothing in the Regulations to limit representation to the official trade union safety representatives. The Commission advise keeping the safety committee 'compact... and compatible with the adequate representation of the interests of management and all the employees including safety representatives'. The other stipulation is that 'the number of management representatives should not exceed the number of employee's representatives'.

Management side representation should be at a very senior level to emphasize the organisation's commitment to health and safety and to add authority to agreed action plans. For a district safety committee it would be appropriate for an authority member to be present together with the DGM, UGMs, the directors of personnel and works and the district nursing adviser.

The staff side members should reflect as widely as possible the workforce in the authority, delegated from and selected by the staff side health and safety representatives. In addition there are likely to be those in each district with particular expertise who may appropriately sit as independent advisers. For example:

— the Occupational Health Service Physician and/or Nursing Adviser

— the Training Officer

— the Principal Medical Laboratory Scientific Officer

— the Fire Prevention Adviser

The Committee should be empowered to co-opt other persons as may service its needs. However, in the process of monitoring the authority's health and safety policy the occupational health department is strategically placed to render assistance and information to the committee, and should be encouraged to do so.

Reporting Injuries, Diseases and Dangerous Occurrences

It is the legal duty of every employer to keep a written record of all notifiable accidents, i.e. all accidents by which an employee is incapacitated for work for more than 3 consecutive days. This record—the Accident Book—is to be kept at the workplace and should be accessible to managers and safety representatives. It provides the employer with valuable information regarding safety at work. However, such accidents are also reported to the HSE. The Regulations apply to employers and the self-employed. The Reporting of Injuries, Diseases and Dangerous Occurrences Regulations (RIDDOR) introduce an altered and expanded system from the previous requirements—the Notification of Accidents and Dangerous Occurrences Regulations, 1980 (NADO). NADO regulations were replaced by RIDDOR on 1 April, 1986. Forms F2508 and F2508A are used for these purposes.

The old NADO regulations required certain particulars of work accidents reported to the DHSS to be sent to the HSE. However, the DHSS/HSE data link was severed by the introduction of the statutory sick pay scheme and resulted in a massive loss of information on accidents and dangerous occurrences at work. The RIDDOR requirements are an enlargement of NADO, simplifying some aspects and aiming to re-establish the data link. Specific injuries are included and the types of injuries which must now be reported have increased. It is important to note that all 'over-three-day' incapacities resulting from injuries at work are now reportable. Under RIDDOR the definition is 'more than three consecutive days excluding the day of the Accident but including any days which would not have been working days.' Days off and rest days therefore count. With this emphasis on accident reporting, it is important to remember that the objective of all safety regulations is to reduce the occurrence of accidents and improve health and safety at work. It is important therefore that adequate feedback of accident information is complemented by appropriate discussion, decision making, and action, leading to tangible improvements. We consider that failure on this point alone is often responsible for a deterioration in staff/management relations and can ultimately lead to a failure in co-operation on the various safety committees, however appropriately they are constituted.

Safety Audits and Safety Inspections

The term 'safety audit' has been subjected to a number of different interpretations. It could be argued that an audit, as in the field of accountancy, aims to disclose the strengths and weaknesses and the main areas of vulnerability or risk, and is carried out by appropriately qualified personnel, including safety professionals. Therefore, a safety audit would subject each area of activity to a systematic critical examination with the object of minimizing hazards. Every component of the total system is included, e.g. management policy, attitudes, training, features of the process and of the design, layout and construction of the plant, operating procedures, emergency plans, including firedrills, personal protection standards, accident records and so forth. An audit would not be carried out more than once per year and a formal report and action plan would be subsequently prepared and monitored.

A safety audit should be carried out by the safety

supervisor and safety representatives, together with a representative of management and a safety adviser. Sometimes, limited audits may be required, say, of fire-fighting appliances. In this case the fire prevention adviser would provide the expertise required. The Fire Brigade are available to advise on the siting of dangerous chemicals and gas cylinders, and the Radiological Protection Supervisor will advise on the use and disposal of radioisotopes, drawing up local rules under the corresponding regulations. Safety inspections are conducted at not more than 3-monthly intervals by the safety representative and safety supervisor within a unit or department. The inspection should check maintenance standards, employee involvement, working practices, rather than the wide-reaching or in-depth approach taken in audit. It is important to recognize that audits and inspections are learning opportunities for both management and workers, and that the principle of discussion and negotiation should be used to resolve differences of opinion that may arise during these activities. We have observed that it is not unusual to find that supervisors will be more likely to criticize working practice and representatives will tend to blame poor equipment for a failure to maintain adequate safety standards. The road to improvement may well lie somewhere between the two and will require negotiating skill and a thorough knowledge of the regulations to resolve the problem. Where the agreed results of a safety audit lead to requests for 'small works' to repair a building failure or to make alterations, it is important to set agreed time limits and to monitor the completion of the work. Such work may well have budgetary implications and agreements reached during an audit must have the backing of the budget holder who will pay for any work required. For this reason the UGM or his senior representative is the most appropriate manager to accompany a safety audit.

The Powers of an Inspector

A Health and Safety Executive Inspector may:

— enter premises at any reasonable time, or at any time in a situation which in his opinion is dangerous

— enquire into all health and safety matters

— demand to see any person

— demand information

— examine, search and make tests

— demand facilities and assistance

— seize and destroy dangerous articles and substances.

In addition, if the inspector is obstructed, he has the power under Section 20 of the HSW Act, 1974 to return accompanied by a police constable. This last power brings home the fact that the Act forms part of our criminal, rather than civil, law. In fact, an inspector may take with him any other person duly authorized by his (the inspector's) enforcing authority together with any necessary equipment or materials that he may need. There may be occasions when an inspector may require the advice of a specialist expert, say, for example, in the field of microbiology, radiation safety or chemical analysis and he is entitled to be accompanied by such persons as necessary.

In practice and in the spirit of the legislation we have found that Inspectors seek to forge co-operative links with management and initially, unless obstructed or confronted with a very serious health and safety situation, will act in the role of advisers and negotiate reasonable time scales for such improvements as they deem necessary. Frequently it is management's reluctance to spend money on improvements that constitutes the 'obstruction' to the inspector and he may then choose to issue a 'notice' in order to direct funds to the required solution. Indeed, such a move may be welcomed by subordinate tiers of management and trade unions alike as an effective lever with which to activate a higher level of decision-making in the organisation in favour of health and safety. An inspector will require to examine the local and departmental safety policies and codes of practice that have been compiled to meet local requirements. He may examine the manager's knowledge of such codes and, if relevant, statutory regulations looking not so much for an ability to recite them, but for an adequate knowledge of their content and application. These might include such matters as the handling of cytotoxic drugs, the Ionizing Radiations Regulations and the disposal arrangements for clinical waste. In addition to managers, subordinate staff may be similarly questioned about actual practices.

The inspector will usually wish to see the workplace, paying particular attention to the main sources of hazard. Where appropriate, a report of his visit will follow with recommendations for improvements. It is common to identify minor points that, while not immediately hazardous, need improvement. Many of these may require 'small works' money, or simply a change in working practice by the staff concerned. The inspector will look for an improvement in these areas no less than in other more serious matters. An inspector's report which only gave a priority list might mean that only the most serious faults received attention. However, the report should indicate those areas that, if his recommendations are neglected, could attract a notice.

Prohibition and Improvement Notices

An inspector can issue a prohibition notice if there is a risk of serious personal injury, to stop the activity giving rise to this risk, until the remedial action specified in the notice has been taken. It can be served on the person undertaking the activity, or on the person in control of it at the time the notice was served.

An inspector can also issue an improvement notice if there is a legal contravention of any of the relevant statutory provisions, to remedy the fault within a specified time. This notice would be served on the person who is deemed to be contravening the legal provisions, or it could be served on any person on whom responsibilities are placed, whether he is an employer, an employee, or a supplier of equipment or materials. Such notices will give reasons explaining why they have been considered necessary and will usually come into effect at the end of the time limit normally allowed for appeals. If an inspector thinks that the risk of serious personal injury is imminent, a prohibition notice may take effect immediately. Under Section 24 of the HSW Act, 1974, a person on whom a notice is served may appeal to an industrial tribunal which has the power to cancel or affirm the notice, or affirm it in a modified form. By appealing against an improvement notice its operation is effectively suspended, but this is not so in the case of prohibition notices, unless the tribunal so directs, and then only from the time when the direction is given. Appeals against these notices are not without risk to the employer since they may well result in an order for costs.

Crown Immunity from Prosecution Under the Act

As we have acknowledged, the cutting edge of this legislation lies in the ability of the HSE to use the Courts to enforce the provisions of the Act by the criminal sanction of unlimited fines and imprisonment for offenders.

However, under Section 48, HSW Act, 1974, it is not possible to bring a prosecution against the Crown. It was therefore equally impossible (until 7 February, 1987) to enforce improvements and prohibition notices against Crown bodies such as health authorities. Although they were exempt, the Department of Health informed health authorities that in any situation where an inspector made it clear that he would have served a notice if the health authority were not a Crown body, the authority should take action to cure the problem as quickly as possible. In fact, the HSE adopted the practice of issuing Crown notices to health authorities, which corresponded to statutory notices, but without legal effect. Although an effective method for enforcement appeared to exist in practice, the perceived force of Crown notices was no greater than any other piece of 'advice' or 'guidance' issued by the department, indeed it may even have been less. A variety of excuses and reasons for delay were used to avoid improving health and safety standards in the NHS and almost all of them related to finance.

In 1984, 19 patients died and 355 patients and staff were taken ill from food poisoning at the Stanley Royd Hospital in Wakefield. It was found that insufficient care had been given to plant and equipment and to the maintenance of sound hygiene practices. Following the report into this unfortunate incident the government decided to lift the immunity from prosecution under the HSW Act, initially from hospital kitchens alone. This seemed barely logical, being analagous to the thinking that lay behind the Health and Morals of Apprentices Act, 1802, to which we referred at the beginning of this study. However, following a Lords amendment, Section 2 of the NHS (Amendment) Act, 1986 contained provision to apply general health and safety legislation to health authorities who can now face prosecution for any breach under the HSW Act. As in private companies, an individual NHS employee would be liable to prosecution if he personally contravened one of the requirements of the Act. But the HSE made it clear that they would only prosecute an individual employee of the NHS in circumstances in which they would have brought a prosecution against an individual employed in the private sector. Therefore, the fact that health authorities were exempt from prosecution did not mean that individual NHS employees were more likely to be prosecuted than they would have been in a private company. An employee would not, for example, have been prosecuted for some failure arising from a shortage of resources which it was not in his power to remedy.

The hospital kitchen example above showed that there was failure at every level of management and this appears not to have been a single example. If, for example, top management is unable to persuade any health authority to release sufficient funds for health and safety improvements, the prosecution of individual officers would have been unlikely to secure that objective when the authority, as the responsible (Crown) body, was itself immune from prosecution under the Act. It is perhaps in circumstances such as these that we may see the new legislation being first applied.

Where then and under what circumstances might a NHS officer be individually prosecuted? In guidance issued in the form of a letter to chairmen of health authorities the HSE stated in 1982 that'... the sort of factors which influence such decisions include the extent to which the matter was clearly one over which the manager concerned had control, the extent of his personal knowledge of the circumstances surrounding the event, the degree to which he failed to take obvious preventive measures, and the amount of any previous advice or warning. On the other hand, officers should know that they will not *be* held legally accountable and hence open to prosecution where they have acted in accordance with the authority's or management's directions on health and safety or where there has been a straightforward error of judgement'. Although it would appear to be a contradiction, the legal requirements of the Act were binding on Health Authorities and Scottish Health Boards, notwithstanding their Crown status which protected them only from prosecution as corporate bodies. In other words, they were breaking the law by failing to observe the provisions of the Act but could not be prosecuted for doing so. It is this anomaly that has been removed by the NHS (Amendment) Act, 1986.

Evaluation

How Well Has the Act Worked?

A major success of the Act is that it extended protection to many of the 8 million workers not previously covered by statute law. Now medicine, education and research, entertainment, sport, cultural activities and some types of catering are all covered by statute for the first time, including the self-employed and those in family businesses. Only domestic service employees in private houses are not covered by the Act. Unfortunately, the volume of legislation has not decreased as was intended by Robens. The preceding legislation such as the Factories Act, and the Offices, Shops and Railway Premises Act, which were to have been progressively phased out, have not yet been repealed. Some of this earlier legislation bears no relation to the modern working environment. The new 'legislation' in the form of the many statutory regulations which have emerged since 1975, is not simpler but more detailed, for example the Code of Practice and the Code of Guidance on First Aid is three times larger than its predecessor.

The Robens intention, reflected in the Act, of less statutory regulation and more use of voluntary codes of practice has, in fact, been reversed, and the voluntary element diminished by the linking of regulations to approved codes of practice, for example, on safety representatives and safety committees.

We doubt whether self-regulation is entirely feasible, bearing in mind the conflicting interests of employers and employees. It would surely depend upon a variety of factors such as financial growth, organisational culture, negotiating tradition and, as in the NHS, the number of trade unions operating in the workplace. In the latter instance self-regulation may be impossible, bearing in mind that different unions may have different policies on health and safety issues and on co-operation with management. Moreover, the Act's reference to trade unions, mandatory safety committees and disclosure of information and so forth could be seen as a move towards industrial democracy. Employers might have thought that the Act would give disproportionate powers to trade unions—especially through safety committees—and that such committees would become a wage bargaining weapon. Indeed, throughout the 1970s, there was a strong governmental tide in favour of increasing industrial democracy culminating in the 1977 publication of the controversial Bullock report and the 1978 White Paper on Industrial Democracy.

Following the general election of 1979 this trend has been notably reversed and we note that the Act, while stipulating that employers set up safety committees if so requested, requires only that they *consult* with them. From our experience we observe this to be the current emphasis. There is, therefore, no duty on employers to reach agreement on safety matters with the unions, a fact not always appreciated by some union representatives, although it would seem prudent for management to do so wherever possible. Despite the fact that the TUC had been pressing for years for mandatory safety committees, not all unions have responded. Many have no full-time safety officers or advisers, and some have rejected the self-regulation principle completely and do not wish to accept any responsibility for health and safety, which they see as the duty of management.

When assessed against the aims of the Robens Committee, Allan Holt, Vice-President of the Institution of Occupational Safety and Health, argues that the Act has failed to achieve its objectives. Apart from the failure of self-regulation, he criticizes inspectors for their reticence in giving definitive advice lest they subsequently be quoted in court, and have their interpretation bound in case law, reducing the Act's intended flexibility of application/He also points out that over half the country's employers have yet to produce a safety policy, that there are insufficient inspectors, and that their reluctance to use the enforcement provisions of the Act has resulted in an attitude of *laissez-faire*. We have already seen how reluctance to prosecute offenders contributed to the inadequacy of earlier health and safety provisions.

We believe there is some truth in this analysis in relation to the Health Service. In such situations the real power to influence events, i.e. to call in the Health and Safety Inspectorate and to put pressure on top management, lies with the safety representatives and with the unions who are at liberty to do this when their managers may be constrained not to do so. Good relationships and communications between departmental managers and safety representatives can considerably assist the prosecution of an active policy on health and safety and achieve far more than would be likely were the manager acting alone. To this extent we believe the Act has been successful.

From the employer's point of view there will be times when he will need to enforce adherence by workers to his own safety policy and codes of practice. As McIlroy has put it, 'to protect the legitimacy of safety standards and to avoid criminal responsibilities, management will find itself at times invoking discipline where breaches of safety rules occur and, in certain cases, dismissing an obdurate employee who is in breach of his statutory obligations. An employee committing a breach of reasonable safety requirements is committing a breach of Section 7 of the HSW Act—a criminal offence.'

It is not sufficient for employers merely to provide safety equipment. They must insist on such equipment being worn. Where safety equipment is appropriate and comfortable and procedures reasonable, failure to observe a safety code can lead to dismissal in some cases for a first offence without previous warnings. However, the context of these offences is important. If poor safety practice has been previously endorsed by an organisation, it is unlikely that, in these circumstances, they would be able to defend successfully a plea of unfair dismissal unless verbal and written warnings had first been issued. However, it is recognized that 'there are activities in which the degree of professional skill which must be required is so high and the potential consequences of the smallest departure from that high standard are so serious that one failure to perform in accordance with the safety standards is enough to justify dismissal'. The reader may be able to think of examples within the Health Service where this might be so.

It is important that safety equipment provided for employees should be adequate, comfortable and reasonable to wear. Employees who complain about inadequacies or faults in safety equipment should be taken seriously as the law will not look favourably on managers who sack workers for not wearing inadequate or unsafe equipment. On the other hand, if standards and equipment are adequate then the employee cannot demand more. This may present a difficulty of a different kind in that workers may decide to refuse to undertake a hazardous procedure unless provided with safety clothing and equipment in excess of that prescribed in the regulations. The statutory regulations may also be exceedingly detailed as with the Ionising Radiation Regulations, 1985. The sheer weight and complexity of these regulations may cause undue alarm and some workers may find their perceptions of danger unjustifiably enhanced rather than logically reassured by the resulting local rules. To resolve such fears and avoid the risk of a dispute, the radiation protection supervisor will require, knowledge, sensitivity and skill in drafting and agreeing local rules and initiating staff training to ensure that both complement each other in the position of staff safety. Such a balance of views calls for management to pay attention to detail in its health and safety arrangements and to seek to reach agreement with safety representatives as far as possible. What the law requires, and seeks to maintain, are safe systems of work rather than slavish obedience to rigid and formal codes which have been 'handed down' by management.

Unsatisfactory standards then cannot be enforced by law. Standards and rules should be agreed jointly with the unions involved, widely publicized and referred to in the disciplinary procedure. Breaches of these rules, like any other disciplinary matter, require thorough investigation with dismissal as a last resort.

The HSW Act, 1974 came out of a period of increasing awareness of environmental issues and of relatively prosperous times. We may legitimately ask if we can still afford it? Initially we believe that some organisations over-reacted and established elaborate and expensive health and safety procedures—perhaps through the boardroom fear of 'individual liability'. We hasten to add that we have seen no such reaction in the NHS. Now the subject has settled down and health and safety is not such a prominent issue, the Act and various Regulations having been 'run-in' with a considerable amount of case law interpretation. In industry there is perhaps now a recognition that the cost of safety may be critical for economic viability and thus job security. While industrial accidents and disease can unfavourably affect the ratio of costs to profits it is being recognized that there is required to be an economic interpretation of the term 'reasonably practicable' and to equate the cost of safety with the probability of risk. This kind of analysis is applicable equally to the private and public sector.

Henderson, developing an idea discussed by Robens, explores the feasibility of an injury tax in the form of an increased National Insurance contribution from firms with high incidence of accidents and industrial disease. By taxing the safety output (injuries and disease) of an organisation, one may derive a more appropriate level of safety practice than by laying down (expensive) input standards in the form of statutory safety regulations.

An example of output analysis with respect to a particular code of practice—the Howie Code—is discussed by Cohen. In this paper he describes the prevention of laboratory-acquired infection in terms of both working practice and investment in expensive equipment. He argues that the incidence of disease among medical laboratory workers is no higher, and in some cases lower, than the general population so that while the upgrading of all clinical laboratories to Howie standards would undoubtedly reduce risk of infection to laboratory workers, this is insufficient reason in itself to implement the code. The level of safety chosen ought to be decided on the basis of weighing costs against benefits. Of course, the risks involved in certain aspects of health and safety encountered in health care are not yet fully established but that should not be allowed to detract from the mode of analysis. Such an approach may be well worth investigating since it is likely to allow more voluntary and flexible systems of work to meet local needs than at present obtain. Such has been the increase in prescribed safety methodology since the Act passed into law that normal professional standards are considered insufficient for the maintenance of health and safety. When professionals are asked collectively to pool their acquired knowledge and wisdom in a single written code of practice to cover all eventualities concerning a particular topic, they err on the side of caution.

The general principles laid down in such codes if rigidly followed without professional and common-sense interpretation, may result in absurdities of bureaucractic dysfunction: for example, suppose a safety code specifies that specimens from patients having a particular disease must be transported in plastic bags. It could well be that at the same time specimens from other patients arguably having a more infectious and, perhaps, more dangerous category of organism, may not be placed in bags because no code yet exists which deals specifically with that particular situation! The reaction by some health workers to the disease AIDS (Acquired Immune Deficiency Syndrome) illustrates this point. We have observed instances where some workers appear to have abandoned their professional training and judgement and have hidden behind the interim guidelines for handling AIDS patients and specimens to an extent that treatment is unnecessarily delayed. When the guidelines were revised, we noticed that attitudes had hardened and fear still inhibited working practice.

Responsibility for some of this defensive attitude may

be fairly attributed to those clinicians who fail to identify high-risk patients or who do so unjustifiably late in treatment. Systems of safety frequently cross organisational boundaries and require commitment from all workers and all occupational groups. A voluntary code may be. difficult to achieve but it is more likely to be followed than one which is imposed, particularly if it is seen to benefit only one type of worker. For example, clinicians and nurses ay believe themselves to be at a high level of personal risk when treating a patient, yet they are obliged to observe what they may regard as unduly time-consuming prro-cedures designed to protect other workers whom they imagine to be at a lower risk, e.g. laboratory workers. As a result some, if not all, of the safety procedures for identifying and transporting high-risk specimens may be overlooked.

It appears to us that the pre-Robens problems of inflexibility have not been solved and that in due time the whole approach to health and safety will require a radical overhaul. Meanwhile, should expenditure on this aspect of health services be reduced, the interpretation of 'reasonably practicable" will be required to place greater emphasis on methodology and technique and less on the purchase of new and expensive equipment.

MISCELLANEOUS POLICIES AT STANFORD HOSPITAL & CLINICS &/OR LUCILE PACKARD CHILDREN'S HOSPITAL

Appointment to the Medical Staff

Before a member of the faculty or staff is permitted to assume responsibility for the care of patients at Stanford Hospital and Clinics and/or Lucile Packard Children's' Hospital, he or she must apply for Medical Staff membership and be approved through a formal credentialing process. In order to avoid delay in beginning patient care, physician candidates for faculty or staff appointments who are expected to manage hospital and/or clinic patients should be assisted by the department to make early application for Medical Staff membership. Information and applications for both Stanford Hospital and Clinics and Lucile Packard Children's Hospital are available at the credentialing office (650) 725-6021.

Requirements for Malpractice Insurance Coverage for New Faculty Physicians & Staff Physicians

Department chairs may wish to keep the numerous required approvals and forms in mind when scheduling the dates on which new faculty physicians and other physicians or psychologists are to begin clinical duties.

Before a new faculty physician, Voluntary Clinical Faculty member or Staff Physician can be provided malpractice insurance and assigned patient care responsibility, the following requirements must be met and forms completed:

- Formal School and/or University (as applicable) approval of the faculty or staff appointment
- Formal approval of a Medical Staff appointment at Stanford Hospital and Clinics and/or Lucile Packard Children's Hospital
- California Medical Licensure form, indicating that the new appointee has a valid California Medical License without encumbrances. Before offering the candidate a position, the department chair should determine that the candidate holds such a license or can obtain one before assuming patient care responsibilities.
- If the candidate is not a US citizen, a completed Exchange Visitor Sponsorship Request form. For

information about the requirements for foreign nationals, contact Bechtel International Center.

— Letter of Agreement on Professional Fees to transmit professional fees to the appropriate Stanford Hospital and Clinics or Lucile Packard Children's Hospital account, signed by the new appointee.

Annual Off-Duty Time in Lieu of Vacation

Members of the Academic Council (University Tenure Line, Nontenure Teaching Line, and Nontenure Research Line faculty) in the School of Medicine are paid for eleven months of service over a twelve-month period from September 1 to August 31. Therefore, during each academic year, the faculty member has a period of one month "off duty." This off-duty time may be taken all at once or in increments throughout the year as determined by the department chair to be consistent with the faculty member's fulfillment of his or her academic responsibilities. The period of one month off duty is not termed "vacation." The unused portion of the month cannot be carried forward into a subsequent year except by prior approval by the department chair of an individual arrangement justified by academic considerations. Pay in lieu of off-duty time or for unused portions of such time at year-end or on termination of appointment is not possible. Medical Center Line faculty are eligible for time off and sabbatical on the same terms as members of the Academic Council.

Family and Medical Leave Policies

Stanford University's family and medical leave policies are more fully described in the *University's Faculty Handbook*. The department submits the signed *Faculty Application for Leave of Absence* form (see below) to the Office of Academic Affairs (OAA), where it is reviewed. The OAA forwards the request to Finance, where it is reviewed in regard to funding.

The Senior Associate Dean for Academic Affairs then reviews the application to determine credibility of the leave plan and notifies the department of the outcome. For additional information, contact the Benefits Office.

Maternity Leave

Maternity leave (disability leave) for a period of time before and after delivery is at full salary. The leave period is determined by the faculty memberís physician, who certifies the number of weeks that she is disabled, both before and after delivery. Partial salary offset is provided by short-term disability insurance for which the woman faculty member is expected to apply. For additional information, contact the Benefits Office. (rev. 11/13/03)

Child Care Leave

Child care leave without salary, normally approved upon request, may be for a mother or a father of an infant for up to one year. Child care, medical, and family care leaves without salary may affect a faculty member's appointment end date.

Delay of Tenure Decision

A one-year extension of the date on which tenure would be automatically conferred is granted upon request to nontenured faculty members who give birth. For faculty appointed prior to September 1, 1996, two such extensions are allowed regardless of whether or not a leave is taken. For faculty appointed September 1, 1996 or later, there is no limit to the number of extensions; however, for these faculty, there is a ten-year limit on the amount of time that may be spent in an untenured rank. These delays do not automatically extend the mother's appointment to the faculty. Her reappointment would be subject to the normal review process including a departmental vote. An additional delay of the tenure decision is granted for the period of leave of absence without salary taken by either the mother or father of an infant (either born to or adopted by parents). The faculty member will automatically receive a reappointment equal to the duration of the leave without the necessity of a departmental review or vote. A parallel rule applies to women in the Medical Center Line. Please contact the Senior Associate Dean for Academic Affairs for further details.

Reduced Teaching Load

Faculty who request this option should not be required to engage in classroom teaching during the quarter in which birth takes place or the following quarter. They should not be required to assume extra burdens of teaching when they resume full-time work in subsequent quarters. Continuation of research, advising and committee duties is expected after the period of maternity leave.

For most women faculty in Clinical Departments, the closest analogy to classroom teaching with respect to time and effort is clinical service. It is the policy of the School of Medicine that a faculty member, on request, will be excused from clinical responsibilities (as well as classroom teaching, if any) for ninety days following the end of her maternity leave. (During maternity leave, the faculty member is not on duty at all; as noted above, the period of maternity leave may be up to four months.) During these first ninety days following the end of maternity leave, the expectation is that she is responsible for her duties other than clinical responsibilities (e.g., continued research and scholarship, student training, committee and departmental work, etc.) and that she will remain on full salary during this time. If the faculty member wishes to return to her clinical responsibilities sooner, she may do so, but this should be a free choice on her part. If advanced planning efforts of the faculty member and department indicate the need temporarily to hire a physician to provide clinical coverage, funds for this purpose will be provided by the Stanford Faculty Practice Plan. Justification for such a request will be required.

Additional relevant sections of the *University's Faculty Handbook* referring to family and medical leave policies are:

— Maternity Leave and Child Care Leave for Ranks in the Tenure Line, Section 2.II.B.2.e. for the possible effect on the tenure clock

— Maternity Leave and Child Care Leave for Ranks in the Research and Teaching Lines, Section 2.II.B for the possible effect on the appointment end date

— Maternity Leave and Child Care Leave for Ranks in the Medical Center Line, Section 2.III.B for the possible effect on the appointment end date

Clinical Faculty Parenting Leave Procedure

Note: This Procedure is in force for requests received for FY 2002 and will be refined for years going forward. Revisions may include a change in the mechanism for collection of the cost recovery and disbursement of the funds through the School of Medicine. Requests prior to FY 2002 will be reviewed and dealt with separately.

Background: In FY 2001, a parenting leave pool in the amount of $200,000 was established for the Clinical Departments using the shared expense methodology on the PSA. The parenting leave pool functions as a shared risk pool. To fund the pool, each department is charged an amount based on the their clinical faculty imputed headcount. The total pool amount will be evaluated annually and changed based on the utilization of funds from the previous year; if funds are left over at the end of the year, the remaining pool dollars will be brought forward to the next year and the parenting leave pool will be reduced accordingly to maintain the desired pool amount. Conversely, if the amount required exceeds the $200,000 pool, the departmental parenting pool allocation will be increased accordingly.

Procedure: Per School of Medicine Policy (Stanford University Faculty Handbook, faculty may request to be excused from clinical duties (including classroom teaching, if any) in the 90 days after their parenting leave. (Note: Only faculty are eligible for coverage. California allows up to four months for parenting leave). ìFacultyî includes male faculty who become new fathers or adoptive fathers during the 90 days immediately following the arrival of the child. The parenting pool funds are available for the payment of the base salary (as defined by the Schoolís Compensation Plan) of the individual on leave, to cover the clinical time of the faculty member during the entire leave period. Requests for funds should be submitted to the Senior Associate Dean of Finance and Administration for approval, using the attached request form. Requests should be made immediately following the conclusion of the leave period. Oncc approved, the request will be routed to the Controller for the School of Medicine (Perry Everett), for transfer of funds to the department.

Sabbatical Leave Policy

Sabbatical leave policy in the Medical School follows University guidelines as stated in the *University's Faculty Handbook*. The process for application is the same as for family and medical leaves (see above).

Research Grant Applications by Faculty Members with Expiring Appointments

A contractor such as the University has an obligation to disclose to an external granting agency any material facts bearing on the institution's ability to carry out the research programme described in a grant application. Since this obligation is widely understood, Stanford does not have a written policy or procedure specifically addressing it.

However, the Sponsored Projects Office does consistently follow a policy of making such disclosure to the granting agency when the grant application is submitted.

Availability of a proposed principal investigator is a material condition of any research grant or contract awarded to Stanford. Therefore, when a principal investigator's faculty appointment will terminate prior to or during a proposed project's period of performance, the potential sponsor should be so informed by the Sponsored Projects Office.

If the principal investigator or the department chair wishes to discuss the manner in which this information is transmitted to the granting agency, the department chair should call the Sponsored Projects Office before or when the grant application is forwarded to that office.

Principal Investigator Waivers

The role of principal investigator generally cannot be assumed by those with an Acting title. An early PI Waiver may be obtained for any faculty candidate whose appointment file has been read by the Senior Associate Dean for Academic Affairs and for whom the Office of Academic Affairs is willing to support submission of application with the caveat that funds will be accepted only upon final approval of the candidate's faculty appointment. In such an instance, the Research Management Group will obtain this permission directly from the Office of Academic Affairs.

In addition, effective January 31, 1997, there is an option of a blanket PI waiver for individuals with Medical Center Line (MCL) appointments. Only members of the

MCL doing clinical research are eligible for this program. The department chair in consultation with the Dean's Office determines eligibility. After the faculty appointment has been approved, the MCL member will be eligible to submit, through the department Chair, an application to be a Principal Investigator on clinical research grants. The first such submission must be approved by the Senior Associate Dean for Research; subsequently, a revocable blanket waiver may be obtained for further grants that support research that is a natural outgrowth of the MCL faculty member's clinical care and teaching. The request for the blanket waiver must be submitted by the department Chair to the Senior Associate Dean for Research and must include the clinical areas of expertise previously approved for research and the dates of the current faculty appointment. Provided these guidelines are met, no further waivers will be required. Should the MCL faculty member wish to submit proposals outside the previously approved area of clinical expertise, a PI waiver will be required. For additional information, contact the office of the Senior Associate Dean for Research.

Abuse Reporting Requirements

The California Penal Code requires all health practitioners to report immediately suspected cases of child abuse to the appropriate child protective agency and cases of dependent adult and elder abuse to either the Ombudsperson or to a local law enforcement agency (when abuse is alleged to have occurred in a long-term care facility) or to either the county adult protective services agency or to a local law enforcement agency (when abuse is alleged to have occurred elsewhere). Health practitioners must also report cases in which a person is suspected of suffering from any wound or other injury: inflicted by his or her own act; by another where the injury is by means of a knife, firearm or other deadly weapon; or which is the result of assaultive or abusive conduct. Further, any suspicion of abuse by a health facility or community care facility must be reported to both the local police authority and the county health department. The University is required to obtain a signed statement from all physicians new to Stanford and certain other employees that states they have knowledge of abuse reporting requirements. To fulfill the requirements, a standard form to be signed by the new appointee will be sent to the department administrator as soon as the appointment has been approved. The department administrator should promptly return the form, signed by the appointee, to the Senior Associate Dean for Academic Affairs.

Faculty Incentive Fund

The Faculty Incentive Fund is a programme operated by the Provost to provide partial billet or salary support for new faculty appointments that increase the diversity of the faculty. Appointments from groups such as the following may qualify for the Faculty Incentive Fund Program's support:

- African Americans
- Native Americans
- Chicano/Mexican Americans
- Puerto Ricans

In addition, appointments of candidates from other groups, such as Asian Americans and nonminority women, may be considered for Faculty Incentive Fund support, depending upon the effect of such an appointment on the diversity of the faculty. This might include an analysis in which the available empirical information about the relative proportions of that group in the general population and in the pool of new MDs, PhDs or other likely candidates would be considered.

Defense, Indemnification and Representation

Administrative Guide, memo 15.7, states that "Stanford's policy is to indemnify and defend its faculty and staff in compliance with California Labor Code Section 2802. That statute provides as follows:

'An employer shall indemnify his employee for all that the employee necessarily expends or loses in direct consequence of the discharge of his duties as such, or his obedience to the directions of the employer, even though unlawful, unless the employee, at the time of obeying such directions, believed them to be unlawful.'"

This policy is applicable to situations in which a claim is made against a faculty member arising out of the faculty member's performance or his or her job duties.

If in the course of the University's defense of such a claim, a conflict arises between the interests of the faculty member and of the University, the parties should make appropriate efforts to resolve that conflict. Under these circumstances, it may become advisable for the faculty member to arrange for a consultation with an attorney not simultaneously representing the University, such as from a panel compiled by the Office of the General Counsel for this purpose.

For further information concerning such a scenario, or for other information concerning legal matters, contact the Office of the General Counsel at (650)-723-9611.

Statement on the Respectful Workplace

Stanford University School of Medicine is committed to providing a work environment that is conducive to teaching and learning, research, the practice of medicine and patient care. Stanford's special purposes in this regard depend on a shared commitment among all members of the community to respect each person's worth and dignity. Because of their roles within the School of Medicine, faculty members, in particular, are expected to treat all members of the Stanford community with civility, respect and courtesy and with an awareness of the potential impact of their behavior on staff, students and other faculty members.

5

Aspects of Hospital and Laboratory Safety

LABORATORY SAFETY PLAN

Purpose

This Laboratory Safety Plan (LSP) describes policies, procedures, equipment, personal protective equipment and work practices that are capable of protecting employees from the health hazards in laboratories. This Plan is intended to meet the requirements of both the federal Laboratory Safety Standard, formally known as "Occupational Exposure to Hazardous Chemicals in Laboratories", a copy of which is found in this study, and the Minnesota Employee Right To Know Act (MERTKA). This LSP is intended to safely limit laboratory workers' exposure to OSHA- and MERTKA-regulated substances. Laboratory workers must not be exposed to substances in excess of the permissible exposure limits (PEL) specified in OSHA rule 29 CFR 1910, Subpart Z, Toxic and Hazardous Substances. PELs for regulated substances are provided. PELs refer to airborne concentrations of substances and are averaged over an eight-hour day. A few substances also have "action levels". Action levels are air concentrations below the PEL which nevertheless require that certain actions such as medical surveillance and workplace monitoring take place.

MERTKA requires employers to evaluate their workplaces for the presence of hazardous substances, harmful physical agents, and infectious agents and to provide training to employees concerning those substances or agents to which employees may be exposed. Written information on agents must be readily accessible to employees or their representatives. Employees have a conditional right to refuse to work if assigned to work in an unsafe or unhealthful manner with a hazardous substance, harmful physical agent or infectious agent. Labeling requirements for containers of hazardous substances and equipment or work areas that generate harmful physical agents are also included in MERTKA.

An employee's workplace exposure to any regulated substance must be monitored if there is reason to believe that the exposure will exceed an action level or a PEL. If exposures to any regulated substance routinely exceed an action level or permissible exposure level there must also be employee medical exposure surveillance.

Scope and Application

RSO's – note and delete: In this section, specify which college or department or division is covered by this Laboratory Safety Plan. Also include a list of Principal Investigators, the locations of their laboratories, and a phrase describing of the type of research occurring in that area. The Laboratory Safety Standard applies where 'laboratory use' of hazardous chemicals occurs. Laboratory use of hazardous chemicals means handling or use of such chemicals in which all of the following conditions are met:

(i) the handling or use of chemicals occurs on a 'laboratory scale', that is, the work involves containers which can easily and safely be manipulated by one person,

(ii) multiple chemical procedures or chemical substances are used, and

(iii) protective laboratory practices and equipment are available and in common use to minimize the potential for employee exposures to hazardous chemicals.

At a minimum, this definition covers employees (including student employees, technicians, supervisors, lead researchers and physicians) who use chemicals in teaching, research and clinical laboratories at the University of Minnesota. Certain non-traditional laboratory settings may be included under this standard at the option of individual departments within the University. Also, it is the policy of the University that laboratory students, while not legally covered under this standard, will be given training commensurate with the level of hazard associated with their laboratory work. This standard does not apply to laboratories whose function is to produce commercial quantities of material. Also, where the use of hazardous chemicals provides no potential for employee exposure, such as in procedures using chemically impregnated test media and commercially prepared test kits, this standard will not apply. The researchers listed in the following table are covered by this Laboratory Safety Plan.

Coordination With Other Standards and Guidelines

RSO's note and delete: Several other University standards and state and federal rules pertain to activities carried out in research laboratories at the University. Ask each PI to check the regulations listed, and contact EHS for more information on any standard that may apply to the laboratory operations. The Laboratory Safety Standard and MERTKA address occupational safety issues. Other federal, state and local standards that address use of hazardous chemicals and other materials. Note particularly the listed chemicals with individual standards in the 'Federal' column, since these compounds generally have *action limits* (usually set at half the TLV), *air monitoring requirements*, and *medical monitoring requirements.* If a researcher is using one of these chemicals, or in the unlikely event that there is a conflict between provisions of various standards, the Department of Environmental Health and Safety should be contacted.

Responsibilities

RSO's – note and delete: Tailor this section, identifying by name the administrators, deans, department heads, research safety officers, etc. who have responsibility for the unit covered in the Laboratory Safety Plan (as identified in Section 1.B. Scope and Application). Implementation of the Laboratory Safety Standard at the University is a shared responsibility. Employees, supervisors, Research Safety Officers, department heads, deans, upper administrative staff, and DEHS staff all have roles to play. These roles are outlined below.

(a) President, Vice Presidents, Provosts and Chancellors (Central Administration)

Upper level administrators are responsible for:

- promoting the importance of safety in all activities;
- promoting the same attitude among all levels of employment at the University;
- supporting a broad-based laboratory safety/chemical hygiene program that will protect U of MN laboratory employees from health effects associated with hazardous chemical, physical or biological agents; and
- ensuring that deans, directors and department heads provide adequate time and recognition for employees who are given laboratory safety responsibilities.

Performance will be measured by:

— DEHS's documentation and annual reporting of the level of compliance within each of the reporting units.

(b) Deans, Directors and Department Heads

DDDs are responsible for:

— identifying at least one technically-qualified research safety officer for the unit. (Colleges or institutes that are made up of a number of large laboratory-based departments are urged to assign research safety officers within each department. Large departments may assign one research safety officer for each division);

— transmitting the name of the designated research safety officer to the U of MN's Chemical Hygiene Officer;

— ensuring that the designated research safety officer is adequately trained regarding the roles and responsibilities of the position;

— ensuring that the designated research safety officer modifies this generic Laboratory Safety Plan to incorporate location-specific information;

— ensuring that the designated research safety officer reviews and evaluates the tailored LSP at least annually, and submits a copy of the modified plan to the Chemical Hygiene Officer for approval;

— taking appropriate measures to assure that college/department/division activities comply with University and OSHA laboratory safety policies;

Performance will be measured by:

— DEHS's record of a trained, research safety officer for the unit.

— DEHS's record of a current, tailored Laboratory Safety Plan for the unit.

(c) Department of Environmental Health and Safety (DEHS)

The Chemical Hygiene Officer for the University is Dawn Errede, and the entire DEHS staff will participate in providing resources for departments in the development of their individual health and safety programs. The Department of Environmental Health and Safety is responsible for:

— preparing and updating the University's generic Laboratory Safety Plan;

— distributing the LSP to departments or other units who will tailor and implement the plan;

— training designated departmental research safety officers regarding compliance with the laboratory safety standard;

— monitoring the progress of departments toward achieving compliance.

Performance will be measured by

— DEHS's documentation that review and evaluation of the generic LSP occurs at least annually, updates as necessary;

— annual feedback to DDDs regarding DEHS's records of lab safety officer training and current LSP s within the units;

(d) Research Safety Officer

The RSO's Roles and Responsibilities are described in greater detail in the RSO Toolkit (http://www.dehs.umn.edu/training/rso/roles.shtml). Briefly, the RSO will:

— serve as liaison between employing department and the Department of Environmental Health and Safety;

— know the rules, to help researchers comply with applicable state, federal and university requirements;

— develop and implement a Laboratory Safety Plan for the department;

— coordinate training to ensure all researchers understand their responsibilities and the policies that apply to their research.

— coordinate inspections of laboratories and ensure laboratory supervisors address any noted deficiencies;

— keep records to document compliance with state, federal and university requirements.

Performance will be measured by DEHS's documentation that:

— review and evaluation of the tailored LSP occurs at least annually;

— the research safety officer's personal training records are current.

(e) Supervisors/Principal Investigators

The immediate supervisor of a laboratory employee is responsible for:

— assuring that potential hazards of specific projects have been identified and addressed before work is started;

— ensuring there are written, laboratory-specific standard operating procedures for the protocols carried out in the laboratory that incorporate directions about how to mitigate the hazards of the procedures.

— informing and training employees regarding the specific hazards in their area and in the work they will be doing;

- scheduling time for the employee to attend designated training sessions;
- enforcing U of MN safety policies and safe work practices;
- conducting periodic audits of the research space under the supervisors control;
- reporting hazardous conditions to the college or departmental research safety officer;
- investigate laboratory accidents and send an Accident Investigation Worksheet with recommendations to the departmental research safety officer for review.

Performance will be measured by:

- home department's documentation of current, pertinent safety training for the supervisor and each employee in the supervisor's group;
- home department's documentation of regular audits for laboratory space under the control of the supervisor.

Employee

Employees who have significant responsibility for directing their own laboratory work are responsible for assuring that potential hazards of specific projects have been identified and addressed before work is started. All laboratory employees however, are responsible for:

- attending safety training sessions;
- following safety guidelines applicable to the procedures being carried out;
- assuring that required safety precautions are in place before work is started; and
- reporting hazardous conditions as they are discovered.

Performance will be measured by:

— supervisor's assessment of employee's adherence to topics covered in safety training.

LABORATORY AND X-RAY PROCEDURES

Laboratory codes have nuances that may promote confusion. Most codes for specific analyte/method and specimen source/analyte combinations have been eliminated. The rheumatologist must be certain that the correct code is applied to ensure proper reimbursement. Offices that process laboratory tests should follow the guidelines listed below:

1. If you do the testing in your own laboratory, bill for the test using the appropriate laboratory code number, in addition to the office visit.
2. If you collect the specimen and send it to an outside laboratory, bill for the office visit and a handling fee (CPT codes 99000-99002) or add the modifier "-90" (or the five-digit modifier 09990) with the code for the test performed. This alerts third-party payors that an outside laboratory performed the tests and supports the billing by both the rheumatologist and the laboratory.
3. If the laboratory bills you for the tests, bill the patient using the appropriate code from the laboratory section. *This applies only to non-Medicare patients. Medicare patients who have laboratory tests performed by an outside laboratory must be billed directly by the outside laboratory*. It should be pointed out that, at least in a few states, Medicaid and other third-party payors stipulate the same requirements.
4. If you are unable to locate a specific code for a test

in the AMA CPT manual, try to find it based on the method of performing the test. Refer to subsection information under the guidelines for the Pathology and Laboratory section.

5. The allowable laboratory tests reimbursed for particular diagnoses are carefully monitored. You should consult your Medicare carrier's bulletin to identify the laboratory tests that will be reimbursed only if it corresponds with the medically necessary diagnosis list.

Blood Counts

Not only are there codes for manual and automated performances of complete blood counts, there are also codes for each component. Refer to the index in the AMA CPT manual for the appropriate list of codes. For most single or small group offices, the codes for hematocrit (CPT 85014), colorimetric hemoglobin (CPT 85018), platelet count (CPT 85590) and automated hemogram (CPT 85021-85027) may be the ones most frequently applied. It is recommended that your billing form list those tests that regularly apply to your practice.

Urinalyses

Urinalyses (CPT 81000-81005) can be listed as a complete routine (with pH, specific gravity, protein, reducing substance and microscopy) or by constituent subsets (complete microscopy) or qualitative chemical analysis with any number of constituents.

Cultures

Body fluids cultures may be described using CPT codes 87001-87999, depending on the site or origin and the type of culture obtained. Urine cultures are usually performed in a quantitative manner with colony counts. Use CPT

87087 if the test was performed with a commercial kit, CPT 87086 if it was done by another method and CPT 87088 for organism identification in addition to the culture codes themselves.

Organ or Disease Oriented Panels

Lab panels have undergone significant changes in the past few years, and they remain a source of confusion. There is no longer a list of automated multichannel tests. Tests should be reported individually unless they comprise one of the 12 organ or disease oriented panels. Physicians should not order one of the organ or disease oriented panels simply as a convenience. If medical necessity is not present for even one of the tests on a panel, then the panel should be "broken" and the medically necessary tests reported individually. HCFA maintains lists of appropriate diagnosis codes for each lab test. If you order a test that is not on the list of approved tests for the diagnosis code(s) you have listed for the patient, you will likely not receive payment for the test. You should contact your Medicare carrier for the approved lists of ICD-9 codes for each test you routinely order. In many cases, carriers have removed the non-specific or unspecified diagnosis codes from the approved lists. You may need to make an educated guess of a specific diagnosis based on information in the file, your physical findings or conversations with the referring physician. Keep in mind that it is fraudulent to list a diagnosis that is not present so that a test will be covered. But, it is not fraudulent to make a specific diagnosis based on your non-lab findings and then change the diagnosis if the labwork does not support your earlier conclusion.

Arthritis Panel

The arthritis panel has four tests: uric acid, blood, chemical (CPT 84550); sedimentation rate, erythrocyte, nonautomated (CPT 85651); fluorescent antibody, screen, each antibody (CPT 86255); and rheumatoid factor, qualitative (CPT 86430). If you order all four of these tests together, you can report a single CPT code, 80072. If individual tests are ordered in addition to a panel, the specific codes for these tests should be reported separately in addition to the panel code. Refer to the AMA CPT manual for a complete list of the appropriate codes. These tests include, but are not limited to, erythrocyte sedimentation rate, synovial fluid analysis, complete blood count (CBC), fecal occult blood test, urinalysis, rheumatoid factor screen, spun microhematocrit, antinuclear antibodies (ANA), complement antigen, complement functional activity, anti-DNA and anti-DNA titer. What many rheumatologists may not know is that there is a code to describe rheumatoid titer (CPT 86431), as well as rheumatoid factor (CPT 86430). Tissue typing can be coded as a single antigen, e.g., HLA-B27 (CPT 86812) or multiple antigens (CPT 86813). A separate code is utilized for HLA-DR/DQ typing, with codes for single antigen (CPT 86816) and for multiple antigens (CPT 86817). Separate codes for complement C3 and complement C4 have been deleted. If reporting C3 and C4 during the same visit, use CPT 86160 and indicate two units under 24 G (Days or Units) on the HCFA 1500 claim form. There is a separate CPT code, 86162, for CH50. If coding for an individual complement (i.e., C2), use CPT 86160 also.

Synovial Fluid Examination

Synovial fluid examinations should be coded as follows:

1. Gross examination (CPT 85810)
   - Viscosity
   - Color
   - Clarity

2. Cell count
   - Total white cell count (CPT 89050)
   - Total white cell count plus differential (89051)
   - Polarizing light microscopy for crystal identification (89060)
3. Glucose (CPT 82947) (list the body fluid being analysed in the narrative field)

Drug Monitoring

Medicare carefully monitors follow-up testing. Listing disease-specific diagnosis codes will not be sufficient to prove medical necessity for drug monitoring. You must also list the ICD-9-CM codes that support medical necessity for high-risk medications. These include:

> V58.69 Long-term (current) use of other (high-risk) medications.
>
> V67.51 Following completed treatment with high-risk medications.

The following table from *Arthritis & Rheumatism* outlines monitoring strategies for methotrexate treatment and should serve as the basis for laboratory testing.

A. Baseline

1. Tests for all patients
   - (a) Liver blood tests (aspartate aminotransferase (AST), alanine aminotransferase (ALT), alkaline phosphatase, albumin, billrubin), hepatitis B and C serologic studies
   - (b) Other standard tests, including complete blood cell count and serum creatinine
2. Pretreatment liver biopsy (Menghini suction-type needle) only for patients with:
   - (a) Prior excessive alcohol consumption

(b) Persistently abnormal baseline AST values
(c) Chronic hepatitis B or C infection

B. Monitor AST, ALT, albumin at 4-8 week intervals

C. Perform liver biopsy if:

1. Five of nine determinations of AST within a given 12-month interval (6 of 12 if tests are performed monthly) are abnormal (defined as an elevation above the upper limit of normal).
2. There is a decrease in serum albumin below the normal range (in the setting of well-controlled RA)

D. If results of liver biopsy are:

1. Roenigk grade I, II or IIIA, resume MTX and monitor as in B, C1 and C2 above
2. Roenigk grade IIIB or IV, discontinue MTX

E. Discontinue MTX in patient with persistent liver test abnormalities, as defined in C1 and C2 above, who refuses liver biopsy

Source: Kremer JM, Alarcon GS, Lightfoot, Jr RW, Willkens RF, Furst DE, Williams JH, Dent PB, Weinblatt ME: *Methotrexate for Rheumatoid Arthritis: Suggested Guidelines for Monitoring Liver Toxicity.* Arth Rheum 37,3,1994, 316-328

Radiologic Examination

As with laboratory codes, several codes are available for each radiologic examination depending on the number of views obtained. To ensure proper reimbursement, the correct code reflecting the total number of procedures performed should be chosen. The use of the modifier "-50" or 09950 should be used to indicate bilateral radiographs. Specific codes for radiologic tests (single and multiple views) can be found in the AMA CPT manual.

There are several CPT codes for bone densitometry. Dual energy x-ray absortiometry (DEXA) has separate codes for axial (76075) and peripheral (76076) scans. Ultrasound bone density scans should be reported using code 76977.

A word of caution is offered here regarding patients covered by Medicare. If radiologic studies are personally performed by the physician or by the physician's employees under appropriate supervision and that physician provides the interpretation, the radiologic studies may be billed routinely as a global service (both technical and professional component). If, however, a radiologic study is obtained that the physician did not actually perform or supervise, then billing and reimbursement fall under the "purchased service" provision. The purchased service may by billed directly to the Medicare carrier by the provider of the technical component, or the physician can bill for it. If the physician bills for it, he or she must check "Yes" in Block 20 of the claim to indicate the technical component was purchased and indicate the actual amount paid for the service. In addition, a "Yes" requires completion of Block 32 with the name, address and Medicare billing number of the provider providing the purchased service. A "No" in Block 20 tells the Medicare carrier that there are no purchased services on the claim.

Certain procedures, including many radiographs and bone density scans, are a combination of a professional and technical services. Use of the modifier "-26" with these codes indicates that only the professional service (interpreting the data) was provided. The modifier "-26" is used by rheumatologists who provide a written interpretation on a radiograph or bone density scan from an outside laboratory. Rheumatologists who only review a radiograph from an outside laboratory and do not provide written interpretation would not use modifier "-26" as this work is considered part of the E/M service.

If a rheumatologist performs or supervises a radiograph in the office and provides written interpretation, then the usual radiologic procedure code, such as CPT 73100, is used. If another physician requests a report on a film done elsewhere, then CPT 76140 (consultation on radiographic examination made elsewhere, written report) is used. A written report is required. This code is not applicable when the physician requesting the report is from the same institution or practice.

U OF MN DEPARTMENT OF STANDARD OPERATING PROCEDURES

RSOs note and delete: Subsections 1, 2, and 3 present the topic headings for the detailed Standard Operating Procedures already included in Appendices D, E, and F. Ask PI's to review these subsections and appendices and train staff on all the SOPs which pertain to the chemicals and procedures used in the laboratory. Work with particularly hazardous or unique chemicals and/or procedures may not be covered by the SOPs listed below. In this case, the PI must ensure the researchers follow written SOPs that describe the work to be conducted, and the safety measures to mitigate any hazards. Procedures and written safety precautions included in laboratory notebooks may serve as laboratory-specific SOPs. Ensure the PI's keep these individual SOPs in the laboratory and train employees on their contents. Ask the PIs to forward a list of these SOPs to the you so they can be referenced in subsection 5 of this chapter.

As noted, Principal Investigators are responsible for ensuring there are written standard operating procedures (SOPs) for the research protocols conducted in their area.

The SOPs must identify the hazards of the protocol, as well as measures to be taken to mitigate those hazards. The references listed below may provide enough detail to serve as the SOPs for some research protocols. Others

Chemical Procedures

A. Prudent Practices in the Laboratory

Laboratory standard operating procedures found in Prudent Practices in the Laboratory: Handling and Disposal of Chemicals (National Research Council, 1995) are adopted for general use at the University of Minnesota. Departmental Research Safety Officers have hard copies of this text, and the entire contents are accessible on the web. Note especially the following topics which are covered of Prudent Practices:

Working with Chemicals

- — Introduction
- — Prudent Planning
- — General Procedures for Working with Hazardous Chemicals
- — Working with Substances of High Toxicity
- — Working with Biohazardous and Radioactive Materials
- — Working with Flammable Chemicals
- — Working with Highly Reactive or Explosive Chemicals
- — Working with Compressed Gases

Working with Laboratory Equipment

- — Introduction
- — Working with Water-Cooled Equipment
- — Working with Electrically Powered Laboratory Equipment
- — Working with Compressed Gases

— Working with High/Low Pressures and Temperatures
— Using Personal Protective, Safety, and Emergency Equipment
— Emergency Procedures

B. The American Chemical Society's "Safety in Academic Chemistry Laboratories"

ACS's "Safety in Academic Chemistry Laboratories" another useful text. This manual presents information similar to that found in Prudent Practices, but in a considerably condensed format.

C. Hazardous Waste Management

Extensive and detailed policies regarding hazardous waste management are specified in the University's guidebook "Hazardous Chemical Waste Management, 5th edition". Please refer to this text for approved waste handling procedures.

D. Emergency Procedures for Chemical Spills

The procedures listed below are intended as a resource for your department in preparing for emergencies before they happen. If you are currently experiencing an emergency such as a chemical or blood spill, please contact the Department of Environmental Health and Safety at 612-626-6002. Complete spill response procedures are described in the Hazardous Chemical Waste Management guidebook (http://www.dehs.umn.edu/guidebook/guidebook3.html). However, the quick reference guide is included for convenience in this Laboratory Safety Plan.

Quick Reference Guide

Evacuate

— Leave the spill area; alert others in the area and direct/assist them in leaving.

— Without endangering yourself: remove victims to fresh air, remove contaminated clothing and flush contaminated skin and eyes with water for 15 minutes. If anyone has been injured or exposed to toxic chemicals or chemical vapors, call 911 and seek medical attention immediately.

Confine

— Close doors and isolate the area. Prevent people from entering spill area.

Report

— From a safe place, call the Department of Environmental Health and Safety (EHS) (612) 626-6002 during working hours, 911 after hours (Twin Cities Campus 911 operators will contact on-call EHS personnel).

— Report that this is an emergency and give your name, phone and location; location of the spill; the name and amount of material spilled; extent of injuries; safest route to the spill.

— Stay by that phone, EHS will advise you as soon as possible.

— EHS or the Fire Department will clean up or stabilize spills, which are considered high hazard (fire, health or reactivity hazard). In the case of a small spill and low hazard situation, EHS will advise you on what precautions and protective equipment to use.

Secure

— Until emergency response personnel arrive: block off the areas leading to the spill, lock doors, post signs and warning tape, and alert others of the spill.

— Post staff by commonly used entrances to the area to direct people to use other routes.

After an accident, supervisor(s) must complete and fax in reporting forms within 24 hours. Workers' Compensation policy and reporting forms are available on the web.

2. Biohazardous Procedures

At the University of Minnesota, researchers must follow the policies in the CDC/NIH text, Biosafety in Microbiological and Biomedical Laboratories, 4th Edition, May 1999. A copy of this text is available on the web at http://bmbl.od.nih.gov/. Another useful reference is the National Research Council's text "Biosafety in the Laboratory: Prudent Practices for Handling and Disposal of Infectious Materials" (1989), available on the web at http://books.nap.edu/books/0309039754/html/R1.html#pagetop. In addition, researchers working with biological materials must acquaint themselves with the policies of the university's Institutional Biosafety Committee (IBC), which are on the web at http://www.ibc.umn.edu/homepg.html. The IBC is charged under Federal Regulations and Regents' Policy with the oversight of all teaching and research activities involving:

- Recombinant DNA
- Artificial Gene Transfer
- Infectious Agents (bacteria, viruses, protozoans, fungi, etc.)
- Biologically Derived Toxins

If the research involves work with any of 31 infectious agents or 12 biological toxins (federally designated as Select Agents), follow the procedures outlined in the Select Agent section of the IBC Web page (http://www.ibc.umn.edu/select.html).

3. Radioactive Procedures

All researchers using radioactive materials at the University of Minnesota must:

— contact the Radiation Protection Division;

— obtain a permit for the possession and use of radioactive materials;

— complete required training modules; and

— comply with the radiation policies and procedures of the university (contained in the Radiation Protection manual).

The Radiation Protection manual contains information on a number of topics including license committees, the permitting process, purchasing procedures, transfer procedures, general safety, personnel dosimetry, waste management, emergency management (spill control), record keeping, and regulatory guides (declared pregnancy workers, risks from ionizing radiation exposure).

Initial training is required for all personnel who are authorized to access radiation areas. Training tapes can be viewed in Minneapolis in the Learning Resources Center (LRC) at the Biomedical Library in Diehl Hall, in the St. Paul Library LRC, and at the UMD Library LRC. After viewing the tapes, users fill out a questionnaire and then recieve specific, on-site training required by permit holder (trainer).

General Safety Procedures

Other University of Minnesota Policies for Safe Practices in Laboratories are accessible in this laboratory safety plan.

Lab Safety

— Emergency Eyewash and Safety Shower Installation

— Eye Protection/Personal Protective Equipment

— Flammable and Combustible Liquid Quantities in U of M Laboratories

- — Controlled Substances
- — Greenhouse Policy-Fumigation/Smoke Generation Procedure
- — Labeling Chemicals
- — Lock Out/Tag Out
- — Respiratory Protection Program
- — Termination of Laboratory Use of Hazardous Materials

Fire Safety

- — Flammable and Combustible Liquid Quantities in U of M Laboratories
- — Fire Safety at the University
- — Portable Fire Extinguishers-Type and Placement

General Safety

- — Emergency Procedures
- — Eye Protection/Personal Protective Equipment
- — Extension Cords in University Buildings
- — Foot Protection/Safety-Toe Shoes
- — Holiday Decorations
- — Portable Fire Extinguishers-Type and Placement
- — Public Corridors
- — Respiratory Protection Program
- — Step Ladders-Care and Use
- — Temperature Standard
- — University of Minnesota Twin Cities Campus Smoke-Free Indoor Air Policy
- — Supervisors Injury/Illness Investigation Form
- — Working with PCBs

Laboratory-Specific Standard Operating Procedures

Guidance: In this section, reference any laboratory-specific SOPs that the PIs in the department have developed to cover chemicals and/or procedures not addressed in

Subsections A, B, and C (above). Some departments include these SOPs , and attach a Laboratory Safety Information Sheet to each protocol/procedure. In this section, simply note what specific SOPs have been developed and how employees can access them.

This section summarizes laboratory-specific SOPs. The full text of these SOPs is included in this study, or can be obtained from the referenced PI, or from the research safety officer, [name], for the Department of [name]. Safety information is included in each SOP, and may be highlighted in a Laboratory Safety Information Sheet, similar to the one included in this study.

General Emergency Procedures

The procedures listed below are intended as a resource for your department in preparing for emergencies before they happen. If you are currently experiencing an emergency such as a chemical or blood spill, please contact the Department of Environmental Health and Safety at 612-626-6002. For University employees who have been exposed to bloodborne or other infectious pathogens, please follow the procedures below under "Needle Stick." For all other emergencies call 911.

Campus Safety Information Guidebook (http://www.dem.umn.edu/guidebook/)

— bomb threats

— medical emergencies

— safety on campus

— severe weather

— utility outages

— warning systems/sirens

6

Preventive Health Care: Roles, Responsibilities and Legal Aspects

PREVENTIVE HEALTH CARE

Why is Preventive Health Care So Important?

About half of all deaths from heart disease are sudden and unexpected, so there's little opportunity for treatment. For people at risk of sudden death, prevention is the key. In 2001 an estimated 516,000 coronary artery bypass procedures were performed on 305,000 patients. If all heart attack-prone people were treated surgically, the cost would be prohibitive. Technological treatments for heart disease such as balloon angioplasty, thrombolytic therapy (clot-busting drugs), antiarrhythmic drugs and pacemakers aren't cures. More importantly, such procedures can't slow the buildup of fatty deposits in arteries (atherosclerosis), which causes most heart disease. And because of supply problems and other issues, heart transplants aren't a realistic option for everyone with severe heart disease. That's why more effort must be focused on prevention. Atherosclerosis often begins in childhood, but it may be decades before clinical disease shows up. We don't fully understand all the causes of heart disease, but many population studies have identified major risk factors and strategies to reduce the risk. These are the risk factors we can modify, treat or control:

— tobacco smoke
— high blood cholesterol
— high blood pressure
— physical inactivity
— obesity and overweight
— diabetes mellitus

The decline in death rates from cardiovascular disease in the United States is mainly due largely to the public's adopting more healthful behaviours and lifestyles. This decline underscores why it's important for the medical profession to advocate prevention strategies. More and more evidence shows that fatty plaques in arteries can regress even in people with advanced disease. As our understanding of the causes of heart disease and stroke has improved, the association is directing preventive measures at health care providers, public health practicioners, community leaders, policy makers, patients and families, who can work together to implement our Primary and Secondary Prevention Guidelines. By focusing on prevention, we can have a major impact on people's health. The American Heart Association wants all people to know their risk factors for heart disease and stroke and the goals for both prevention and treatment. This approach includes people knowing how to effectively use the many strategies available to achieve these goals. Prevention costs less than expensive medical interventions, and in the long run brings more benefits.

AHA Scientific Position

The American Heart Association believes that basic preventive health care services should be an integral part of an equitable, comprehensive health care plan, accessible to all. In the past three decades great strides have been made in preventing and treating heart disease and stroke.

Death rates from cardiovascular disease have declined as a result, mainly because so many people have made positive behaviour and lifestyle changes.

Hospital Admission

The most important right of a member of a hospital medical staff is the right to admit patients to the hospital. The admission of a patient of a patient to a hospital requires decisions by both the admitting physician and the hospital administrator (in the latter case the decisions being usually delegated to an admitting clerk). The interaction of these two decision makers may have serious consequences that must be considered in the medical quality control program. The most common conflict arises when the admitting clerk declines to admit a patient that the physician has ordered to be admitted. The usual reason is that the patient is unable to pay for the hospitalization. If the planned treatment is strictly elective, the physician will usually cancel the admission until the hospital's financial criteria have been met. At this point, assuming that the patient has no preexisting relationship with the hospital, the patient has no cause of action against the hospital's refusal of admission. However, the physician may have a cause of action against the hospital for interfering with the physician's practice, the damages being the fees lost through the hospital's refusal to admit the patient. If the admission is not strictly elective, the hospital's position is more precarious. The hospital administration cannot admit patients to the hospital; this privilege is limited to the members of the medical staff. While a veto by the administration over an admission is not exactly the same as an administrative decision to admit a patient, the result is the same: the administration has substituted its opinion for the physician's opinion. The legal question is whether anyone is injured by the veto. In the elective admission, the patient may suffer an injury by having the admission delayed. The physician's cause of action will still include the economic interest but will also include an action for indemnity if the hospital refusal of the patient causes the physician to be sued for malpractice. If the physician classifies the admission as an emergency, the hospital is obliged to admit the patient. Refusing an emergency admission will result in almost certain liability if the patient is injured by the delay. This liability stems from the combination of the impermissible exercise of medical judgment by the administrator and the duty to render emergency care when the emergency is known and the physician has accepted the patient. The quality control manager must ensure that the admitting clerk does not turn away a patient without immediately informing the treating physician. The bylaws or section rules should provide a procedure for the physician to contest the refusal of admission, including the right to demand that the patient be admitted unless a medical reason is shown why the patient was refused admission and the time when the physician is able to have the patient admitted elsewhere.

Discharge Records

The physician's discharge order and follow-up care instructions should also be entered into the medical record. The discharge note should contain any pertinent medical findings and the discharge dictation should be done promptly. The physician should be careful to record in the medical record, as well as in the patient's office chart, all outpatient prescriptions given the patient. The medical record must reflect the patient's condition at the time of discharge, including the reasons for follow-up care. There is a temptation to put very little information in the chart at the time of discharge and then put the necessary, more complete information in the dictated discharge summary. While not ideal, this is acceptable if the discharge summary is done at once. Unfortunately, discharge summaries are often put off until weeks or months later. The physician's memory is not fresh at the point, so the discharge summary must be reconstructed from the chart. If all the necessary information is not in the chart, the accuracy of the discharge summary may be questioned. Additionally, if the patient suffers an adverse consequence before the discharge summary is dictated, the discharge summary will be questioned as being self-serving to the extend that it relates exculpatory information not otherwise documented in the chart.

Discharged from the Hospital

Just as a hospital administrator cannot admit a patient to the hospital, the administrator cannot discharge a patient from the hospital. A patient can be discharged from the hospital only by a physician. The physician may issue a discharge order when the patient is able to continue convalescence without further medical care. The patient who needs only minor additional care may be discharged with instructions to return to the physician's office (or the emergency room) for follow-up care. The physician is responsible for the patient's condition upon discharge and will be liable for any injuries suffered from a premature discharge. The physician is also responsible for either personally providing or personally arranging follow-up medical care. The instructions for follow-up care should be clear and should be written out and given to the patient.

Release Forms

If the physician is unable to persuade the patient, or if the patient seems unwilling to wait for the physician, the hospital administrator should discuss with the patient the decision to leave. In many cases, the patient may have valid complaints that can provide valuable information to the quality control manager. Irrespective of the reason, if the patient still insists on leaving, most hospitals will try to persuade the patient to sign a release of liability, colloquially called an "against medical advice" (AMA) form. The AMA form typically states that the patient was warned of the risks of leaving the hospital prematurely and waives any cause of action against the health care provider. This type of waiver, called a blanket release, is ineffective in court because public policy prohibits releasing a person from liability for negligence. The only value of this form is as evidence that the patient was warned about the risks of leaving the hospital. Unfortunately, the release section in the form causes many patients to refuse to sign it. A better approach is to use a questionnaire-type, elective discharge form that provides information about the patient's complaints and details the risk that we told to the patient. This form should not contain any release of liability; this will increase the chances of its acceptance by the patients. The legal value of the questionnaire form is that it delineates the patient's complaints. The hospital may offer to correct any legitimate problems and will be alerted to any misunderstandings that need to be documented in the medical record. If the patient later sues on a new complaint, the hospital will be able to document that it was never notified of the problem and thus had no opportunity to correct it. This will also diminish the patient's credibility as a witness because of the conflicting complaints. In effect, a properly designed elective discharge form has the legal standing of a statement by the patient, rather than the appearance of a coerced release. The courts will look on this much more favorably than they do the usual AMA form.

Bill Payments

Another possible false imprisonment situation occurs when the hospital gives the patient the impression that the patient cannot leave the hospital until arrangements have been made to pay the hospital bill. This is especially risky when the patient is a minor and the parents are unaware of their right to take the child. This situation usually arises from the actions of an overzealous billing office employee. the hospital administration is seldom aware that the billing office tries to intimidate patients into making arrangements for the bill before leaving the hospital. This is usually discovered only after a lawsuit is brought for false imprisonment because a child was left in the hospital for a few days by distraught parents who did not know that they had the right to take their child home. The billing office personnel must be made aware of this problem; there should be prominent signs in the billing office explaining that the patient (or parent) may leave when discharged. Giving the patients this information will also decrease the likelihood that payment contracts signed by the patients will be attacked in court as coercive.

LSU LAW CENTER'S: MEDICAL AND PUBLIC HEALTH LAW SITE

Management Control

The basis of management control theory, are used in this book, is the concept of the control loop. A simple example of a control loop is that of a loading dock attendant using hand signs to help a truck driver park at the dock. In this case, the attendant is the manager, the truck driver is the person (actor) responsible for carrying out the task, and parking the truck is the task. For each action taken by the driver, the dock attendant evaluates the outcome (position of the truck), compares that outcome with the desired outcome (the truck property parked at the dock), decides what corrective action the driver must take, and signals the driver to take the selected corrective action (gives the driver feedback). This sequence is repeated until the truck is docked. The loop is closed when the attendant advises the driver to change direction, and the loop is repeated until the truck is properly docked. If the dock attendant's supervisor watched this process and then told the attendant not to direct the trucks so close to the dock in the future, a second loop would be created between the attendant and the supervisor. Personnel may be involved in multiple control loops, as managers in some loops and actors in other loops.

There are six elements in a control loop:

1. input: the data on which the manger must base selected actions
2. analysis: the manipulations that must be performed on the input before it can be used for decision making
3. decision making: the process of comparing the analyzed data with the appropriate standards to determine if the manager needs to intervene to alter the process being monitored
4. intervention: the action taken by the manager to alter the outcome of the process being monitored
5. evaluation: the comparison of the actual effect of the intervention with the desired effect
6. feedback: the modification of the management strategy based on the evaluation of the effect of the intervention of the outcome of the process

The simplest management control loops, such as the driver-attendant loop, contain only Steps 1 through 4. In this example, Steps 5 and 6 were added when the supervisor became involved in the loop. The driver-attendant-supervisor loop spans three management levels; in a large business the control loops may reach through many levels of management.

The most important consideration in analyzing management control loops is to determine if they are closed.

For a loop to be closed, the manager must be given information about the changes the manager's interventions produce in the actor's performance and the manager must modify the intervention strategy accordingly. If there is no feedback of information about the outcome of the management activities, the manager may engage in counter productive intervention strategies without being aware of their adverse consequences. For example, a hospital administrator might deny patients access to their medical records unless they have a letter from an attorney, without knowing whether this encourages patients to sue the hospital on the assumption that the hospital is covering up something. The nature of control loops is best illustrated through a detailed analysis of their component parts.

State Laws

Health care providers must be especially careful of false imprisonment situations because the courts are allowed to award punitive damages to a falsely imprisoned patient. The only effective defense against a suit for false imprisonment is to rely on relevant state laws about emergency confinement of patients. These laws vary from state to state and should be carefully researched for the state where the facility is located. In general, the state laws on emergency confinement are intended for mentally ill patients and will not protect the hospital for detaining a competent patient. If it is necessary to detain a patient to prevent immediate harm from cessation of medical care, the health care provider may be able to get a court order based on the failure of the patient to understand the situation. The law allows the greatest freedom of action when a temporarily incompetent patient is involved. This is common intensive care units, where a confused patient will pull out the tubes and head for the exit, often stark naked. While restraining such a patient might technically be false imprisonment, it is clear that the hospital would have greater liability if it did not restrain the patient. If there is a valid medical reason for restraining a patient for a short time, the courts are unlikely to consider it a false imprisonment. False imprisonment is likely to be found only when there is no acute harm threatened and the patient is competent. In the unconsented transfer situation, it is likely that a competent patient would be able to maintain a suit for false imprisonment. In this case, there would be a forcible transfer to the ambulance and the holding of the patient in the ambulance. This is legally very different from simply restraining a temporarily incompetent patient. If the patient were unconscious, there would not be any false imprisonment because the patient would not be aware of the limitations on the patient's actions. The situation of an unconscious patient presents other consent problems, but it does not present a false imprisonment problem.

Inappropriate Delegation of Authority

Inappropriate delegation of authority can refer either to the delegation of too much authority or to the delegation of too little. Over delegation of authority is most serious when it results in nonphysicians exercising medical judgment. This can arise either in the process of directly delivering care or during the establishment of administrative rules governing the delivery of health care. The most common direct care problems involve nurses who are put in the position of screening patients' requests to see a physician. These may be patients seeking care at the emergency room or patients on the floor who wish to see a physician. In the first case, the hospital must be careful that no patient is turned away from the emergency room without seeing a physician. Even in states that do not statutorially require the rendering of emergency medical care there can be substantial liability for refusing care in a situation where a patient has relied on the hospital's representation that it offers emergency medical care. This problem can be prevented by logging in each patient on a computer, then using the computer to ensure that the patient is not ignored. The hospitalized patient who requests to see a physician presents a special problem because there is a duty to care for the patient and because a hospital is clearly liable if the nursing staff injures a patient by denying the patient access to a physician. This is an example of the type of problem that must be explicitly addressed in the nursing protocols. As discussed later, a major quality control activity is the reviewing and updating of nursing protocols to eliminate risks. This is not enough, however. There must also be an educational program to ensure that all nursing personnel, especially contract nurses, are aware of all changes in the protocols. This educational function is critical to an effective quality control program, because it ensures that the staff members (both medical and nursing) understand their roles in the quality control program.

The problem of too little delegation of authority arises when questions that require timely answers are reserved for high-level administrators or medical staff committees. If, for example, the decision to admit an emergency patient without insurance is left to the chief administrator, there will be many times when that administrator is unavailable to make the decision. This can create severe legal problems if the administrative delay results in injury to the patient. This problem is exacerbated when the decision is left to a committee, because it is extremely difficult to have committee meetings on short notice. It is thus essential to ensure that all decisions that must be made in a timely manner are not dependent upon personnel who may be unavailable. The quality control program should always be structured as a "fail-safe" system, in which the inability to find the proper person to make a decision will not interfere with the rendering of needed medical care.

Broken Line of Command

Broken lines of command occur when a task or decision is routed to a person or committee that either does not act on it or does not propose appropriate interventions. An example would be an infection control program that compiled statistics on the patterns of infection but did not attempt to change the protocols for handling infectious diseases. Another example would be a medical staff committee that did not take action on complaints against staff members. Such a committee would "break" the control loop by not proceeding to the intervention step. In this case, the broken loop would have serious legal implications, because it would be simple to demonstrate that the failure to take action against the errant physician was due to negligence by the oversight committee.

Historical Perspectives

The first hospitals were founded in the Middle Ages. The only similarity between these facilities and the modern hospital is that they both house sick people. The hospital in the Middle Ages was run by the Church as a way station between this life and the next. While a patient would be fed and clothed, it was considered an evil act to attempt to cure the patient 's illness. Sickness was a manifestation of God's will, and it was not up to human to change God's will. In contrast, the modern hospital sees its role as that of providing acute care medical services intended to cure the patient's illness.

Several hundred years elapsed before hospitals became the "physician's workshops" that we are familiar with. The transition was complicated by the continuing involvement of religious orders, especially nuns, in the building and running of hospitals. This involvement created a tension between the spiritual orientation of the hospital and the secular nature of modern medicine. The nuns were seen as reverent and self-sacrificing, the physicians as materialistic (the accuracy of these stereotypes is irrelevant to their impact upon the law). This perception resulted in a reluctance to allow lawsuits against hospitals because the court viewed these suits as being against the self-sacrificing nuns who ran the hospital. The questions was seen as a choice between compensating one injured patient or providing care to many sick persons. Since the hospital (viewed as a charity) retained no earnings, a judgment against the hospital would have been borned by the poor that the hospital served. The accuracy of these perceptions notwithstanding, the law solidified into the doctrine of charitable immunity. This doctrine prevented a patient from suing a hospital if the patient was injured in the hospital. This immunity from suit has disappeared over the last 15 years, but it still influences the way hospitals view their legal responsibilities. The fundamental expression of its influence is the assumption that the interests of the medical staff are the same as the interests of the hospital. As the rationale for hospitals shifted from rendering spiritual aid to rendering medical services, the medical staff became the most powerful group in the hospital. The physicians often helped to finance the original construction of the hospital and were essential to its survival. Nonmonetary considerations also bolstered the physician's power.

One of the classic distinctions between physicians and hospital personnel has been sex. Physicians were men; hospital personnel, whether nurses or nun administrators, were women. The physicians traveled in the same social circle as the members of the hospital board of trustees. The hospital personnel, whether men or women, were poorly paid and did not interact with the board of trustees except in the employer/employee relationship. An administrator or nurse who displeased a physician could expect to be fired. This led to the attitude among early hospital administrators that their job was to serve the needs of the medical staff, an attitude that created the concept of the hospital as a "physician's workshop." The physicians workshop theory holds that a hospital has no direct relationship with the patient. The only provider-patient relationship is between the patient and the physician. The hospital may provide nursing personnel, but these nurses provide care only under the supervision of the physician.

In the same way, the physician is held responsible for ensuring that all of the equipment provided by the hospital is in proper working order. This is clearly an unrealistic view of the modern hospital; it is doubtful that it was even an accurate portrayal of the 19th century hospital. This type of unrealistic theory is called a legal fiction. A legal fiction usually exists to remedy a defect in the law that would otherwise lead to injustice.

The injustice that the fiction of the physician's workshop addresses stems from the charitable immunity bar to litigation. The courts are very reluctant to deny an injured person a legal remedy for the injury. Thus, a person who was injured through the negligence of a hospital employee would be denied any legal recourse unless the courts created a theory to circumvent the doctrine of charitable immunity. One analysis of hospitals during the period of charitable immunity showed that the physicians controlled hospital policies and were the prime economic beneficiaries of the hospital. Since a goal of tort law is to shift the burden of economic loss from the injured party to the person who caused the injury, the court used the borrowed servant doctrine to hold the physicians liable for the actions of the hospital employees.

The borrowed servant doctrine is based on the idea that an employee can be "borrowed" by someone other than the employer. The person who "borrows" the employee becomes liable for the employee's actions. This shift in responsibility for the employee's negligence follows the shift in the responsibility for directing the employee's actions. The employer's liability for the employee's negligence is based on the employer's duty to direct and supervise the employee's job performance. The financial relationship between the employer and the employee does not, in itself, make the employer liable for the employee's negligence. When a person "borrows" the employee and assumes the duty to direct and supervise that employee's activities, the borrower also assume the liability for the consequences of the employee's actions. The courts made the assumption that the physicians had assumed the duty of directing and supervising the hospital employees. This assumption allowed a patient who was injured by a negligent hospital employee to sue the patient's attending physician for the injury. The borrowed servant doctrine was also applied in situations where some of the borrowed servants were not hospital employees. The significant example of this extension was in the operating room. Here the surgeon might be assisted by medical students, residents, and even free-lance operating room technicians.

Since the borrowed servant doctrine was thought of as applying only to employees, the courts created the broader captain-of-the-ship doctrine. This doctrine is based on the assumption that the surgeon directs and supervises the actions of all members of the surgical team. The court analogized this to the role of a ship captain who is responsible for the actions of all members of the crew. (Ship captains are usually sued as the servants of the ship owners, making this analogy more literary than legal.) Like the borrowed servant doctrine, the effect of the captain-of-the-ship doctrine was to give the patient a responsible party to sue. Though legal fictions, both of these doctrines were closed enough to the reality of the times to be reasonable approaches. The reasonableness of the two doctrines has become less clear with the evolution of the modern hospital and the concomitant development of high technology medicine. Four fundamental changes in the practice of medicine led to the abandonment of the physician's workshop type of hospital. The first was the development of multiphysician health care teams. These teams diminished the powerful role of the attending physician, making the hospital personnel responsible to several physicians for direction in the care of a patient. This forced the hospital to assume the responsibility for keeping track of the orders of the entire physician team. Once this responsibility was assumed, it was only a short time before all the administrative aspects of patient care were shifted to the hospital.

The second change was the development of hospital-based physician groups who did not maintain individual practices. These groups formed radiology department, anesthesia departments, clinical laboratories, and other specialty service departments. While such groups maintain the legal facade of private practitioners who perform only contract work with the hospital, this is not a fair picture of their relationship with the hospital. From the patient's point of view these groups are as much a part of the hospital as the nursing service. While only a few courts have held hospitals directly liable for the actions of such in-house physician groups, their existence has caused the courts to increase the hospital's duty to coordinate the medical care rendered to patients.

The third change in medical practice has been the recognition of nursing as a skilled profession. This has been due partly to the increased legal status of women in society and partly to the complexity of nursing tasks in a high technology medical environment. As medical care has focused on (and created, as a result of the increased use of surgery) the critically ill patient, nurses have been called on to make medical judgments. In many critical care situations, the nurses must institute care before a physician can be summoned. Even in noncrisis situations, nurses are asked to perform complex patient care tasks, such as the maintenance of airways and the administration of toxic drugs. Nurses have become autonomous members of the health care team, following physicians' orders but also planning and initiating complex nursing tasks. The need to supervise these self-initiated nursing tasks has required hospitals to develop structured nursing departments that believe the notion of nurses acting only as the borrowed servants of the medical staff. The fourth change has been the growth of proprietary hospitals and hospital management companies. Once hospitals began to be seen as profit-making businesses, the rationale for charitable immunity vanished. (Some courts allowed suits against for-profit hospitals while still barring suits against charitable hospitals.) The changes in medical care delivery have forced hospital personnel to become independent members of the health care team. At the same time, the religious-affiliation hospitals saw the supply of nuns dry up, resulting in all but a few administrators becoming secular employees. Religious hospitals have now become multimillion -dollar enterprises that bear little resemblance to their charitable predecessors. Few of them admit charity patients, and all compete openly against the for-profit hospitals. The courts have responded to this change in mission by ending the charitable immunity doctrine. It is now possible for an injured patient to sue and recover from hospitals without being forced to resort to the legal fictions of borrowed servant or captain of the ship.

Hospital Liability

The liability of an institution for the actions of employees, contractors, visitors, and trespassers is not unique to hospitals. hmos, clinics, group practices, and even individual providers may be held liable in the same way. These providers are especially vulnerable to this type of litigation because they do not have the protection of extensive quality control programs. All health care providers should carefully consider whether, and to what extent, they are involved in the types of legal relationships that may make them vulnerable to malpractice litigation.

The Medical Staff

The liability of the hospital for the actions of a medical staff member flows from the duty to ensure the competence of the medical staff. Except in employment or agency situations, the hospital is not directly liable for the negligent actions of a medical staff member. For example, if a nurse gives a patient the wrong medicine, the hospital would be liable for the mistake. However, if a physician gives a patient the wrong medicine, the hospital would not be liable unless it was negligent in allowing the physician to have (or continue to have) staff privileges.

The granting of staff privileges could be ruled negligent for one of three reasons: (1) the criteria that were used to evaluate the applicant were insufficient to determine the applicant's competence; (2) the hospital board knew that the physician was incompetent; or (3) the board should have known that the physician was incompetent. The third situation, "should have known," is narrowly defined. It usually refers to circumstances where the nursing or the medical staffs were aware that the physician was having trouble. The board members can be put on notice of misbehavior by the reports of staff members or on the basis of their personal knowledge or information from an outside source, such as patient complaints. A failure to act when the board members have personal knowledge of negligent behavior could, as noted earlier, result in personal as well as corporate liability. The breach of the initial duty to screen applicants for basic medical abilities is seldom sufficient to support a malpractice judgment. The failure must be obvious to reach the level of negligence. The board is allowed nonphysicians to be called doctor and to write medication orders on patients. A more common problem involves a failure to check the references be checked. A hospital that fails to discover that an applicant lost privileges elsewhere could be liable to patients injured by that physician.

Failing to discipline a physician for acts of negligence or bad judgment is the best-established basis for a suit based on negligent entrustment. If the hospital is to avoid liability, the board must act when it knows of wrongdoing. The chance of a board member being held personally liable is remote at this time, but rapid changes are being made in this area of the law. Lawsuits based on negligent entrustment are a very serious problem. One bad physician can injure many patients, all of whom are potential plaintiffs. If the suits go to trial, the jury may be enraged by the hospital's failure to discipline the physician, despite knowing about the physician's outrageous conduct. From the public relations point of view, this type of incident can affect the reputation of the entire medical staff.

The issue of when the board "should have known" about the physician's misconduct is most difficult to resolve. The courts must balance liability for actions that the board did not know about against allowing the hospital to escape liability by ignoring its duty to oversee the medical staff.

The board must avoid the temptation not to find out what is happening in the hospital. In a self-insured facility, the potential losses from lawsuits by a group of injured patients could be devastating. The amount in a self-insurance trust is based on past experience of the facility and other like it. The calculations assume a relatively steady, fairly random, occurrence of claims. A grossly negligent physician could generate a unpredictable string of claims that could greatly exceed the amount in the trust. (Even conventional insurance has limits on the total claims paid during a given period.) Successful long-term planning must include ways to monitor the performance of the medical and nursing staff. But detecting wrongdoing is only the first step. The hospital must also be prepared to intervene to remedy the problem. Intervention is politically difficult, but a failure to intervene will open the way for malpractice litigation.

The most difficult situation to deal with is that involving a physician who is rendering dangerous care. The critical issue is to provide substitute care for the physician's patients. This is a problem separate from that of disciplining a negligent physician. The hospital bylaws must provide a procedure for the temporary suspension of privileges and the provision of transitional care. This is a drastic remedy, but without it the hospital may not be able to protect patients adequately from negligent injuries. There must also be a provision for the emergency review of privileges. All suspensions should be reviewed by a physician committee, but there must also be a provision for emergency suspension by the hospital administrator. An obvious case would be a physician who comes to the hospital intoxicated. Intoxication sufficient to impair the physician's judgment would be obvious to the nursing personnel. The administrator must be able to suspend this physician's privileges temporarily. Once the nursing staff is aware that a physician is impaired, either by illness or drugs, the hospital will become liable for the physician's actions. Suspending the physician's privileges will satisfy the hospital's obligation to remove the physician.

The emergency suspension of a physician's privileges creates a special problem between the hospital and the patient. In a teaching hospital, where the patients have many primary physicians (or, in the view of some critics, no primary physician), the problem can be easily handled by diplomatically shifting the burden the care to another staff member. Suspension of privileges is also fairly simple in HMOs, where the responsibility for the patient's care is shared by many physicians. However, these two situations are exceptional. In most cases, the primary relationship is between the patient and the physician. The patient seeks care from the physician, who then admits the patient to the hospital. The patient would be justifiably upset to find that the treating physician has lost hospital privileges. The patient's wish, or even demand, to be treated by the physician does not obviate the hospital's liability for any injury that may occur as a result of the physician's negligence.

The inability of the patient's wishes to absolve the hospital from liability has two roots. The first root is the public policy that a person should not assume the risk of the consequences of negligence. This prohibition is necessary because of the unequal bargaining position of the parties in most health care transactions. In the medical situation, a patient often has little choice of physicians during an acute illness. The physician would, of course, like to have the patient agree not to sue if the care is unsuccessful. If the patient could be asked to absolve the physician of liability for negligent actions, society would lose a major control mechanism over the quality of medical care. The patient would suffer by having to choose between receiving medical care with no recourse for a negligent injury or not receiving the medical care. These problems have been weighed (by the courts) against the right of the patient to contract freely with the physician. The courts have ruled that, since the parties seldom have equal bargaining power (one party is not free to reject the unsatisfactory contract) and because the private enforcement assumption of the risk of negligence in the medical contract.

The second root is the hospital's duty to ensure the qualification of its medical staff. In the situation discussed here, the emergency suspension of privileges, the hospital is clearly on notice that the physician is impaired. The hospital's duty to monitor the medical staff is a nondelegable duty. The patient cannot be allowed to assume the responsibility for judging the physician's capabilities. In the same sense, the patient cannot be asked to bear the burden of a hospital's door with a nonstaff physician, the hospital (except in certain emergency circumstances) would not allow that physician to admit the patient to the hospital. In this situation, the hospital's duty is to protect the patient from improper care. The problem is the same if the patient is already hospitalized. If the hospital has notice that the physician is impaired, it has a duty to suspend that physician's privileges.

Once the decision to suspend privileges has been made, the physician's patients must be notified at once. The matter should be discussed with the patients, who should be asked if they want to be treated by another medical staff member. If the patient and another staff member are agreeable, new consent forms can be signed, and the responsibility of caring for the patient can be transferred. The person who talks with the patient—either another medical staff member or an administrator (unless there is a nurse the patient especially trusts)—should be careful to explain that the physician has been incapacitated by an illness or accident and can no longer care for patients. It is not necessary to elaborate on the possible hazards of allowing the physician to continue practicing. The patient who refuses the substitution of a new physician—either in the case of an absent physician or a physician on emergency suspension—is a special problem. The hospital cannot discharge a patient who needs care. A medical staff committee should determine if it is medically appropriate to discharge the patient from the hospital. If it is appropriate to discharge the patient, this will solve the problem of substituting physicians. If it is not appropriate, the hospital must balance its duty to care for the patient against the patient's right to choose a physician. In almost all situations, the patient will eventually allow the substitution of physicians if the matter is carefully discussed so that the patient understands that it is in the patient's best interest. This may require the chief of the medical staff or the chief administrator to spend time with the patient, but this situation is rare enough that it merits such an effort. An alternative is to have the impaired physician appoint someone to take over that physician's patient care duties. While the patient may be dissatisfied with the assignment, it is legally acceptable for a physician to arrange for another physician (with appropriate privileges) to cover the former's practice. If the hospital bylaws specify that all members of the medical staff must designate someone to care for their patient's when they are unable to, the problem of physician substitution will be lessened.

The Hospital Board

The legal structure of a hospital is the same as that of any corporation. There is a board that oversees the overall operation of the facility, officers that carry on the day-to-day business of the corporation, and front-line employees who carry out the orders of the of officers. If the hospital is a for-profit institution, the board is called a board of directors;

if the hospital is a nonprofit, it is called a board of trustees. The duty of the board is to select the officers of the hospital, make policy decisions, and monitor the management of the hospital to ensure that the board's policy decisions are being carried out. If the hospital is private, the board owes its allegiance to the stockholders, who have the right to remove the board if they are not satisfied with its performance. If the hospital is nonprofit, the board owes a duty to the general public. In most states, the only person with standing to challenge the board of a nonprofit hospital is the attorney general. However, since the attorney general seldom has enough resources to monitor trustees, a board of trustees may have more freedom of action than a board of directors.

The liability of the board is synonymous with the liability of the hospital—with limited exceptions. The liability for the actions of all persons for whom the courts may hold the hospital responsible flows to the board, and thus to the corporation itself. There are two situations where the actions of the board are not charged to the corporation. The first is when the board acts in a way that is prohibited by the rules of the corporation(either by the bylaws or by the articles of incorporation) or acts illegally. These actions are termed ultra vires and do not bind the corporation. If the actions harm anyone, the board members themselves may be sued and held individually liable for damages. The second situation involves certain transactions that, while not illegal or specifically forbidden by the corporation rules, are not in the interests of the corporation. This does not apply to simple, bad business decisions; it usually involves a director or trustee abusing a duty to the corporation by making a deal that is personally rewarding at the expense of the corporation.

Board members may be held personally liable if they

neglect their duty to the corporation. An example of this would be a refusal to dismiss a staff member whom the board knows to be guilty of severe misconduct. The hospital would be liable for the misconduct, and the board members could be sued individually for dereliction of their duty to supervise the hospital operations. While most cases involve personal knowledge of the wrongdoing, the law may hold the board members liable if they should have known of the wrongdoing. This prevents the board from avoiding liability by not inquiring into potential misconduct. When the hospital corporation is first formed, all of the rights and duties of the corporation are vested in the board. The board may then delegate certain duties to employee or medical staff committees. The board still retains the responsibility for these tasks and can be held liable if the tasks are improperly performed.

Since the board must delegate most tasks in order to function effectively, its primary function becomes the supervision of these tasks. When the supervision involves employees, the hospital board functions much like other corporate boards. It is in the supervision of medical staff members that a hospital board deviates most significantly from the usual corporate pattern. While many corporations are involved in the supervision of highly trained professionals, only hospitals delegate the task entirely to the professional group. The hospital board must formally approve all medical staff committees decisions, but the board seldom attempts to evaluate independently the committees' decisions. The most important of these decisions is the granting and reviewing of medical staff privileges.

Administrative Actions

The acts of administrative personnel are attributed to the hospital because these workers are directly under the control of the senior staff of the hospital. The hospital can be held liable for the following types of actions by administrators:

— intentional acts that harm patients
— negligent acts that directly harm patients
— negligent supervision of employees or medical staff members that results in patient injuries
— failure to comply with laws governing the reporting and management of public health diseases and violent injuries

Intentionally harmful acts, while rare, pose a special legal problem. The person doing the act would clearly be personally liable for any resulting injuries. The legal question is whether the hospital would be liable for actions that were not part of the person's duties as an employee. The degree of the hospital's liability depends on the foreseeability of the actions. While the hospital would have some liability for any harm to the patient, this becomes more important if the hospital should have anticipated the actions. If the hospital does not screen employees for potential mental problems or past episodes of aberrant behavior, its failure to do so would be a serious breach of the duty owed the patient.

Negligent acts that directly harm patients usually involve decisions by administrators that affect health care delivery to a specific patient, as opposed to policy decisions that may influence the care of all patients. Legally, the most dangerous acts are those that involve medical decision making. Administrative personnel are not permitted to direct either physicians or nurses in any activities that require the exercise of their respective professional judgments. If the administrator is expected to supervise the details of a nurse's work, that administrator must be a properly licensed nurse with a professional standing that is at least equal to that of the nurse being supervised. The administrator who is expected to supervise the delivery of physician services must be a licensed physician with hospital staff privileges appropriate to the actions being supervised. The most common situation in which administrative personnel become involved in medical decision making is in deciding whether a patient will be admitted or treated by the hospital or clinic. The admission of a patient to a hospital is an act of medical judgment. This decision is made by members of the medical staff. However, in most facilities, administrative personnel review the decision through a determination of whether the patient has sufficient resources to pay the hospital bill. This puts the administrator in the position of being able to veto the admission of the patient. If a patient's admission is denied, there could be liability for any harm that results from the denial. In most cases, the decision to hospitalize a patient is an elective decision, and delaying the admission will not harm the patient.

The problem then shifts to the admitting physician. The physician may delay the admission until the patient can raise a deposit, may send the patient to a charity hospital, or may demand that the hospital reconsider its decision and admit the patient. If the physician chooses to either delay the admission or send the patient elsewhere, the hospital is absolved of its responsibility for the patient; the physician will be liable for any injury that the delay causes. However, by ratifying the hospital's decision not to admit the patient, the physician has reassumed the responsibility for the decision. If the physician chooses to demand that the patient be admitted, the hospital must either admit the patient or accept the responsibility for any harm that results from the denial of medical care. This is a difficult position to defend. The only acceptable ground for an administrative decision to deny a patient admission to the hospital is that there is not enough room for the patient or that the patient would pose a physical threat to the other patients. If the hospital relies on one of these grounds, it must be careful to document the exact circumstances of the refusal to admit the patient.

If the refusal is based on the patient's inability to pay (or other nonmedical criteria), the hospital must be able to document that the patient's condition did not require immediate hospitalization. To do this, the administrator must find a member of the medical staff who is willing to examine the patient and determine the seriousness of the patient's condition. If the physician is willing to certify that the patient is not in need of immediate hospitalization, the liability for delaying the patient's admission will shift from the hospital to the physician. In the absence of this second opinion, the hospital has no defensible course other than to admit the patient. The central problem in allowing administrative personnel to make (or veto) medical decisions is that there is no effective legal defense if the decision is wrong. A physician who makes an incorrect decision can present testimony by other physicians to show that the decision was reasonable under the circumstances. The administrator is not allowed this defense because it is illegal for anyone other than a properly licensed physician to make a medical treatment decision. The administrator is limited to establishing that the mistake was not the proximate cause of the patient's injuries.

The most important area of liability for administrative decisions is in the establishment and maintenance of hospital protocols. These may be infection control protocols, incident reporting protocols, or any other protocols that influence the quality of medical care services. If a patient is injured because a protocol is negligently drafted or enforced, the hospital will be liable for any patient's injuries resulting from the negligence. As previously noted, there must be cooperation between the hospital administration and the nursing and medical staffs if the hospital protocols are to be effective. The administration must ensure that all proposed protocols embody proper professional standards and that all members of the medical and nursing staffs are acquainted with the protocols. The most common violation of the public health laws is the failure of the hospital to ensure that proper reports are made when a reportable condition is treated. Most states require the reporting of gunshot wounds, communicable diseases, venereal diseases, and possible child abuse. These reporting laws create a duty for both the physician and the hospital because the hospital's duty to report is usually independent of the physician's duty. While many of the reporting laws carry only token penalties for a failure to report, their violation can also result in civil liability. This is especially true of the venereal disease and child abuse reporting laws. A health care provider who is in violation of a public health reporting law is considered to be negligent per se. This means that the provider is assumed to have acted negligently and will be liable for damages if the plaintiff can prove that the negligence caused an injury. For example, if a provider suspected that a child under the provider's treatment was suffering from child abuse, in many states the provider would have a duty to report the possible abuse to the authorities. If the provider failed to report the possible abuse and the child was later seriously injured, a representative of the child could sue the provider for negligence.

Another legally significant problem involves the treatment of venereal disease. If the health care provider fails to report a case of syphilis, the provider could be liable to those contacted by the treated person because those persons could be liable to those contacted by the treated person because those persons could have been warned if the disease had been reported. This could be very damaging in the case of a married man seeking to have his syphilis treated clandestinely. If his wife is also infected, there would be a significant chance that any subsequent children would be born with congenital syphilis (a terrible condition with permanent sequelae). In this situation, the wife and child would have a strong cause for action against the provider. This type of liability can result from the violation of any of the laws that protect the public welfare.

Nursing Protocols

The development of comprehensive nursing protocols is basic to a nursing quality control program. Most nursing tasks are carried out at the initiative of the nurses rather than in direct response to a physician order. The physician makes the medical decisions about medications, diet, and so on; but he nurses must fill in the details to ensure that the patient receives comprehensive nursing care. The nursing staff must also ensure that nursing services are rendered if the physician is derelict in writing basic orders. While a careful nursing staff will quickly call this problem to the attention of the attending physician, this can delay the patient's care. Since a principal goal of a legally effective quality control program is to reduce litigation through increased patient satisfaction, the delay poses a problem, since it will;l reduce patient satisfaction even if it does not result in an injury.

Beyond seeing that the patient's basic needs are met, the nursing protocols must spell out how to handle patient safety problems. For example, there should be written guidelines for the use of bed rails. Under the present standard of care for hospitals, the decision on when bed rails are needed is left to the nursing staff, unless there are specific physician orders addressing the issue. The use of bed rails is important because an impaired patient can easily fall out of bed. However, bed rails are also very inconvenient. They prevent an ambulatory patient's sense of well-being because they reinforce the patient's sense of helplessness. These disadvantages mitigate against a policy of always using bed rails to avoid having to exercise discretion. In the case of bed rails, the protocols should be in two parts. First, there should be a list of all types of patients who should have bed rails. These might include postoperative patients, children under eight years of age, all patients in traction, all comatose patients, and so on. The second part of the protocols should give the nurse the authority to use bed rails in any other situation where they seem warranted.

It is important that the nursing staff be encouraged to use their own initiative in preventing patient accidents. An overly rigid protocol can reduce this initiative. It should be emphasized, however, that the nurse's freedoms to innovate extends only to using a safety device when it is not normally required. The nurse is not free to disregard a safety device in a situation that is included on the mandatory list. In the case of bed rails, the nurse could use them on a patient who id not fit one of the delineated categories, but would be forbidden not to use them on a patient in one of the categories.

Nursing protocols often deal with procedures that are matters of medical opinion. A physician may order that a gram of penicillin be given the patient in one liter of 5 percent dextrose. The nurse will decide on the type of intravenous (IV) fluid set to use, the size and type of needle to use, and the location of the vein to be used. These decisions should be part of the nursing protocol. This will not create a problem unless the protocol that is followed is in opposition to a physician's order.

For example, assume the nursing protocol calls for a 10-gauge needle on the IV line. This is a relatively large needle and will allow a rapid flow rate. The physician prescribes a drug that is highly toxic if given too quickly. In order to provide an extra measure of protection against too rapid infusion of the drug, the physician specifies that it be given through a 25-gauge needle. With a needle this small it would be impossible to give the drug too fast. However, instead of following the physician's order, the nurse follows the protocol that calls for a 19-gauge needle. The drug runs through too fast, and the patient suffers an adverse reaction from the inappropriate dose rate. In this case, the hospital would be liable for the patient's injury because it allowed the nurse to substitute the nurse's judgment for the physician's, to the detriment of the patient.

It is important to note that the issue is not whether the nursing protocols invade the "practice of medicine." To be useful, nursing protocols must involve some exercise of medical judgment. The physician expects the nurse to know where to give a shot, which needle and drip rate to use on an IV, when an IV must be changed, and the other "routine" skills of drug administration. Yet these skills are different from how to feed a patient or change a bed. The physician will often modify the protocol on drug administration, yet will seldom, if ever, comment on the way the patient is fed or how the linen is changed.

Thus, it is useful to divide nursing duties into two types: (1) skills such as drug administration that involve medical decision making, and (2) skills such as feeding patients and changing linen that do not require medical decisions. Such a decision will facilitate the development of protocols by the hospital administration. The group of skills that involves medical judgment (such as drug administration) should be considered as "physicians' standing orders" rather than as a part of nursing protocol. In a sense, the physician for these standing orders is the medical staff itself. The drafting of such orders should be done in consultation with the medical staff. If the medical staff decides that a particular provision of the protocol should not be modified by an individual physician, the provisions should be delineated in either the medical staff bylaws or in the specialty section rules. This will shift the problem of a physician who wishes to modify a rule to the medical section and away from the nursing personnel. This will avoid conflicts between the nurses and the treating physician.

An example of this type of problem would be rules governing infection control in the hospital. A hospital needs rules on the isolation of patients with certain infectious diseases and how their nursing care is administered. A physician who does not want an infected patient isolated would create a threat to other patients in the hospital. In many hospitals, the job of enforcing infection control policies is handled by an infection control nurse under nursing system protocols. This is an effective mechanism for handling the problem. However, if the physician writes orders that are contrary to the protocol, the nurses will have to invoke procedures for reviewing physician orders. In this case, the burden is on the hospital (through the medical staff) to justify the challenge to the physician's order. If, however, the infection control protocol are part of the medical section rules or bylaws, the burden of justifying a deviation from the infection control protocol will be on the physician.

The shift in the burden of justifying a deviation from established routine derives from the genesis of the two different sets of rules. The nursing protocols that deal with duties such as feeding patients and changing linens are developed by the nursing supervisors, hospital administrators, and, in some cases, medical staff committees. These protocols tend to be totally internal documents. The nursing supervisors and the nursing staff must be familiar with them, but few members of the medical staff will ever see them. In contrast, if the nursing protocols involving medical decisions are incorporated in the medical staff bylaws or medical section rules, they are assumed to be approved by the entire section or medical staff. The bylaws are distributed to all physicians on the staff, and the section rules are distributed to all physicians on the staff, and the section rules are distributed to all members of the specialty section. The medical staff is charged with knowledge of the bylaws and appropriate section rules. Adherence to the bylaws and rules cannot be inflexibly applied in all cases, but the physician is charged with justifying any deviation from them. If the deviation results in a negligent injury, the physician will be liable. The hospital will be liable only if, as discussed later, it breached its duty to supervise the physician.

Medical School Services

Another area where indemnification would be useful is in the relationship between medical schools and nonuniversity hospitals that are used as teaching hospitals. Past court decisions have usually held the medical school liable for the actions of its students and staff. These decisions usually turned on the close relationship between the students, staff, and the medical school. Since the medical school staff members are also members of the hospital medical staff, the hospital could be held liable if it failed to monitor properly the competence of these medical staff members. The problem is that the hospital is seldom able to evaluate independently the credentials of the members of the teaching staff. The usual agreement between the medical school and the hospital allows the medical school to decide who will be on the teaching staff, and it allows all members of the teaching staff to oversee the teaching in the hospital. In this type of situation, it would be in the hospital's interest to require the medical school to indemnify it against any judgments arising from the negligence of medical school personnel. Since the assets of the medical school would be large enough to pay any judgment, the indemnity would not even require the medical school to carry additional insurance. The benefits to the medical school of having the hospital accept its students is sufficiently important that the potential risk of the agreement would be offset.

This balance of interests is basic to the negotiation of indemnification agreements. The hospital can exact indemnification agreements only if the use of the hospital's resources is sufficiently valuable to offset the potential costs of the agreement to the third party. In a teaching hospital, there are two factors that mitigate the risk to the medical school of indemnifying the hospital. First, hospitals are seldom held liable for the actions of medical students or residents. Second, in the usual malpractice suit involving a teaching hospital, the plaintiff will sue the student, the medical school, and the hospital.

Unless the hospital was in actual control of the student, the hospital will be liable only if it breached its duty to monitor the overall quality of medical care. The hospital can escape liability if it can prove that it did not breach its duty to the patient. The best way to do this is to put all of the blame on the medical school. However, this will seriously compromise the ability of the medical school to defend its actions. It is better for the medical school to risk the potential losses of an indemnification agreement than to force the hospital to aid in making the plaintiff's case. In general, it is the potential infighting between defendants that provides the strongest rationale for indemnification agreements.

Altered Records

The health care provider should not alter the medical record under any circumstances. The hospital must zealously guard its medical records from alterations by physicians or members of the nursing staff. Even an inconsequential alteration will throw the validity of the entire record into question. If an entry must be changed, a single line should be drawn through the entry, taking particular care to make sure that the original entry is clearly legible. The new entry should be written above or next to the old entry, and the date of the new entry, as well as the name of the person making the entry, should be recorded.

The entry must also be signed by that person. Juries are very intolerant of altered medical records; and even innocent mistakes, such as the loss of a few pages of a record, will be construed as an intentional coverup. Under no circumstances should materials such as liquid paper or other opaque liquids be applied to the record in order to correct any entry.

Emergency Room Services

In the emergency room setting, indemnification means that some third person, either the physician or the emergency room service company, contracts with the hospital to pay the hospital for any losses the hospital incurs due to the negligent actions of the emergency room physician. The two requisites for indemnification are (1) that the third party be legally obligated to pay the losses, and (2) that the third party have sufficient assets to cover the potential losses. The third party is usually required to carry insurance to cover any expected losses, although this is not essential if the third party has sufficient liquid (and nonexempt) assets. Indemnification is widely used in business contracts, but it is seldom found in medical services agreements.

Physician Service Companies

Indemnification should also be requested from corporations with which the hospital contracts to provide physician services, such as the staffing of emergency rooms. These physician services agreements are very profitable, putting the hospital in a good position to require indemnification. This indemnification is especially important for third party physician groups because of the inability of the hospital to assess the qualifications of those physicians. The hospital is forced to delegate to the third party provider its duty to select medical staff members, but it cannot delegate its liability if this selection is improperly performed. This leads to the hospital being held liable for the results of decisions that it is unable to participate in. By requiring the physician services corporation to indemnify the hospital against any losses that result from the improper selection of emergency room physicians, the hospital shifts the financial risk of an improper decision to the party that actually made the decision. The benefit to the staffing company is that it is allowed to continue doing business with the hospital and it is protected from the hospital cooperating with the plaintiff. If a hospital contracts directly with physicians to staff its emergency room, it is unlikely to be able to negotiate an effective indemnification agreement with physicians. The physicians will seldom have enough available assets to pay a substantial settlement, and the cost of additional insurance may be prohibitive. The same problem may arise if the hospital rilies on members of its medical staff to provide emergency room coverage. In these cases, the hospital's only course is to require that the physicians carry personal malpractice insurance. While this does not directly protect the hospital from losses, it does ensure that the physician will have an attorney to protect the physician's interests. A physician without any assets or insurance may agree to help the plaintiff make a case against the hospital in return for being let out of the lawsuit. The insurance will also provide assets for the hospital to reach if it decides to sue for common law indemnity for the physician's actions.

Disappearance of Records

The disappearance of the entire medical record is extremely damaging in medical malpractice litigation. The disappearance of the records calls into questions the care rendered the patient and the integrity of the hospital. The hospital must carefully guard its medical records to prevent them from being inadvertently misplaced or stolen by an unscrupulous person. Under no circumstances should the medical record be allowed out the medical records department. If a patient is readmitted to the hospital, the relevant parts of the record (admissions and discharge notes, reports of laboratory tests, and other requested information) should be duplicated, and copies should be sent to the floor to be incorporated in the patient's new medical record. The record of the earlier hospitalization should not be sent to the floor and made the basis of the patient's new records. Physicians should not be allowed to check out medical records and take them away from the medical records department. The medical records department should provide a comfortable, quiet area for physicians.to work on medical records and review charts. Only by enforcing an absolute prohibition on removing records from the medical records area can the medical records administrator prevent the inadvertent loss of a record. If records routinely leave the medical records department, it will be very difficult to guarantee that all the records removed are actually returned to the department. Even if an effective mechanism for checking out the records could be devised, if the physician who checks out the record accidentally loses it, the medical records personnel are in the same position as if the record has been stolen.

Retention of Records

There are few legal requirements on how long medical records must be retained after the patient has been discharged from the hospital. From a risk management point of view, it would be desirable for all records to be retained indefinitely. Unfortunately, this would be economically difficult to justify, so reasonable criteria for the retention of records must be adopted. These criteria should balance the risk management benefit of retaining records against the economic problems associated with storing a large quantity of records that will seldom, if ever, needed.

Misfiling Records

Another problem arises in the misfiling of a record. In facilities that have hundreds of thousands of records, the misfiling of a record may lead to its permanent loss. This is not a problem peculiar to medical records storage. Large libraries face the same problem when books are misspelled book is effectively lost. In order to combat this problem, such facilities hire persons whose only job is to do what is called "reading" the shelves. They systematically begin at one end of the collection and scan the titles and the access numbers of every book in the collection to flag misfiled books. In the case of books, this is a cost-effective procedure. A person need only recover one or two valuable books a day to offset the salary being paid. When it is realized that thousands of titles may be scanned in a day's time, the probability that several misfiled books will be located is very high. It is harder to assess the cost effectiveness of this type of surveillance in a medical records department. First, medical records are not in open stacks, so they are usually filed by skilled personnel. The probability of misfiling a record will be considerably lower than it is in a research library where the patrons often refile books themselves. Second, unless a malpractice suit has already been filed in a given case, there is no clear economic benefit to finding a misplaced file. The risk manager must be very forceful in arguing that, even though there is no direct economic gain in finding a misplaced file, the potential loss from litigation is great enough to justify the periodic scanning of the files to recover misplaced medical records.

Statutory Requirements on Record Keeping

There are some statutory requirements on the keeping of medical records. For example, certain Medicaid/Medicare reimbursement regulations require that the medical records of recipients be available for verification of charges for a five-year period. The most comprehensive federal regulations concerning medical records were promulgated by the Occupational Safety and Health Administration (OSHA) and became effective on 21 August 1980. While these regulations may be modified in view of current court challenges, it is expected that their general provisions will survive. The OSHA regulations affect medical records held by health care providers who either work directly for an employer or who have some type of ongoing relationship with the employer. While the legal definition of an ongoing relationship is not clear, it can be assumed that the OSHA regulations would apply to the situation where the health care provider contracts with the employer to render medical care to the employees. The usual example is a clinic that performs preemployment physicals for a given employer. The following OSHA regulations apply to employees who are exposed to toxic agents:

Exposure or exposed means that an employee is subject to a toxic substance or harmful physical agent in the course of employment through any route of entry (inhalation, ingestion, skin contact or absorption, etc.), and includes past exposure and potential (e.g., accidental or possible) exposure, but does not include situations where the employer can demonstrate that the toxic substance or harmful physical agent is not used, handled, stored, generated, or present in the workplace in any manner different from typical nonoccupations situations. The regulation then defines "toxic substance or harmful physical agent" in such a way as to make the class of covered employees very large—"Toxic substance or harmful physical agent" means any chemical substance, biological agent (bacteria, virus, fungus, etc.), or physical stress (noise, heat, cold, vibration, repetitive motion, ionizing and non-ionizing radiation, hypo- or hyperaric pressure, etc.) which:

(i) is regulated by any federal law or rule due to a hazard to health,

(ii) is listed in the latest printed edition of the National Institute for Occupational Safety and Health (NIOSH) Registry of Toxic Effects of Chemical Substances (RTECS)...

(iii) has yielded positive evidence of an acute or chronic health hazard in human, animal, or other biological testing conducted by, or known to, the employer, or

(iv) has a material safety data sheet available to the employer indicating that the material may pose a hazard to human health.

For OSHA purposes, an employee medical record is defined as any record made by a health care provider (doctor, nurse, therapist, and so forth) or medical technician. It includes the entire medical record, employment and medical questionnaires, records of preemployment physicals, screening tests, and x-rays. The regulations exclude physical specimens unless they are covered by other laws. Records of voluntary help programs, such as drug abuse and alcoholism treatment programs and counseling programs, are excluded from the regulation if the records are kept in a place separate from the normal medical records of the patient. The federal regulations provide that the medical records must be maintained for a least 30 years after the termination of employment. The regulations allow the medical records to be reduced by microfilming or other storage techniques, but x-rays must be maintained in their original form. The retention of the original x-rays is important in this type of record because chronic lung disease is a major problem in occupational health. Using current reproduction techniques, there is really no satisfactory way to reduce an x-ray so that all the original information is retained. As noted later in the section on access to medical records, the regulations also provide detailed provisions for employee access to their own medical records.

Bibliography

Allan EL, Barker KN. Fundamentals of medication error research. *Am J Hosp Pharm* 1990; 47:555-571.

Barker KN, Pearson RE, Hepler CD, Smith WE, Pappas CA. Effect of an automated bedside dispensing machine on medication errors. *Am J Hosp Pharm* 1984; 41:1352-1358.

Bates DW, Boyle DL, Vander Vliet MB, Schneider J, Leape L. Relationship between medication errors and adverse drug events. *J Gen Intern Med* 1995; 10:199-205.

Bates DW, Spell N, Cullen DJ, Burdick E, Laird N, Petersen LA, et al. The costs of adverse drug events in hospitalized patients. Adverse Drug Events Prevention Study Group. *JAMA* 1997; 277:307-311.

Borel JM, Rascati KL. Effect of an automated, nursing unit-based drug-dispensing device on medication errors. *Am J Health Syst Pharm* 1995; 52:1875-1879.

Bowman L, Carlstedt BC, Black CD. Incidence of adverse drug reactions in adult medical inpatients. *Can J Hosp Pharm* 1994; 47:209-216.

Choong PF, Langford AK, Dowsey MM, Santamaria NM. Clinical pathway for fractured neck of femur: a prospective, controlled study *Med J Aust* 2000; 172(9):423-6.

Classen DC, Pestotnik SL, Evans RS, Burke JP. Computerized surveillance of adverse drug events in hospital patients. *JAMA* 1991; 266:2847-2851.

Cullen DJ, Sweitzer BJ, Bates DW, Burdick E, Edmondson A, Leape LL. Preventable adverse drug events in hospitalized patients: a comparative study of intensive care and general care units. *Crit Care Med* 1997; 25:1289-1297.

Dardik A, Williams GM, Minken SL, Perler BA. Impact of a critical pathway on the results of carotid endarterectomy in a tertiary care university hospital: effect of methods on outcome. *J Vasc Surg* 1997; 26:186-92.

Dean B, Barber N. Validity and reliability of observational methods for studying medication administration errors. *Am J Health Syst Pharm* 2001; 58:54-59.

Dean BS, Allan EL, Barber ND, Barker KN. Comparison of medication errors in an American and British hospital. *Am J Health Syst Pharm* 1995; 52:2543-2549.

Department of Health and Human Services. Health care financing administration. Fed Regist. 1997; 62.

Facchinetti NJ, Campbell GM, Jones DP. Evaluating dispensing error detection rates in a hospital pharmacy. *Med Care* 1999; 37:39-43.

Felkey BG, Barker KN. Technology and automation in pharmaceutical care. *J Am Pharm Assoc (Wash)* 1996; NS36:309-314.

Guerrero RM, Nickman NA, Jorgenson JA. Work activities before and after implementation of an automated dispensing system. *Am J Health Syst Pharm* 1996; 53:548-554.

Holmboe ES, Meehan TP, Radford MJ, Wang Y, Marciniak TA, Krumholz HM. Use of critical pathways to improve the care of patients with acute myocardial infarction. *Am J Med* 1999; 107:324-31.

Hutchinson TA, Flegel KM, Kramer MS, Leduc DG, Kong HH. Frequency, severity and risk factors for adverse drug reactions in adult out-patients: a prospective study. *J Chronic Dis* 1986; 39:533-542.

Jenkins MH, Bond CA. The impact of clinical pharmacists on psychiatric patients. *Pharmacotherapy* 1996; 16:708-714.

McDonald CJ. Use of a computer to detect and respond to clinical events: its effect on clinician behavior. *Ann Intern Med* 1976; 84:162-167.

Murray MD. Information technology: the infrastructure for improvements to the medication-use process. *Am J Health Syst Pharm* 2000; 57:565-571.

Ried LD, McKenna DA, Horn JR. Meta-analysis of research on the effect of clinical pharmacokinetics services on therapeutic drug monitoring. *Am J Hosp Pharm* 1989; 46:945-951.

Index

R

S

T

U

W

X